How to Succeed in Medical Research

How to Succeed in Medical Research

A Practical Guide

Robert Foley, MB BCh BAO, MSc, MCh, GradCert (Statistics), MRCS
Specialist Registrar in Radiology
Health Education England Severn
Bristol, UK

Robert Maweni, MB BCh BAO, MCh, MRCS (ENT)
Specialist Registrar in Otorhinolaryngology
Health Education England Thames Valley
Oxford, UK

Shahram Shirazi, MB BCh BAO, BSc, MRCS
Specialist Registrar in General Surgery
Health Education England London & South East
London, UK

Hussein Jaafar, BSc (Biomed), MSc (Neuroscience), PhD (Candidate)
Life Science Consultant
Life Science Dynamics
London, UK

WILEY Blackwell

Registered Office(s)
John Wiley & Sons, Inc., 111 River Street, Hoboken, NJ 07030, USA
John Wiley & Sons Ltd, The Atrium, Southern Gate, Chichester, West Sussex, PO19 8SQ, UK

Editorial Office
9600 Garsington Road, Oxford, OX4 2DQ, UK

For details of our global editorial offices, customer services, and more information about Wiley products visit us at www.wiley.com.

Wiley also publishes its books in a variety of electronic formats and by print-on-demand. Some content that appears in standard print versions of this book may not be available in other formats.

Library of Congress Cataloging-in-Publication Data
Names: Foley, Robert (Robert W.), author. | Maweni, Robert, author. |
    Shirazi, Shahram, author. | Jaafar, Hussein, author.
Title: How to succeed in medical research : a practical guide / Robert
    Foley, Robert Maweni, Shahram Shirazi, Hussein Jaafar.
Description: First edition. | Hoboken, NJ : Wiley-Blackwell, 2021. |
    Includes bibliographical references and index.
Identifiers: LCCN 2020045110 (print) | LCCN 2020045111 (ebook) | ISBN
    9781119645498 (paperback) | ISBN 9781119645474 (adobe pdf) | ISBN
    9781119645573 (epub)
Subjects: MESH: Biomedical Research | Research Design | Ethics, Research |
    Research Report | Medical Writing
Classification: LCC R852 (print) | LCC R852 (ebook) | NLM W 20.5 | DDC
    610.72–dc23
LC record available at https://lccn.loc.gov/2020045110
LC ebook record available at https://lccn.loc.gov/2020045111

Cover Design: Wiley
Cover Image: © TECHDESIGNWORK/Getty images

Set in 9.5/12pt Minion Pro by SPi Global, Pondicherry, India
Printed and bound by CPI Group (UK) Ltd, Croydon, CR0 4YY

10 9 8 7 6 5 4 3 2 1

Contents

Foreword

P. Ronan O'Connell

It is a great pleasure to write a foreword for a book written by one's former students, even more so when the theme is *How to Succeed in Medical Research: A Practical Guide.* The authors kindly acknowledge the support and mentorship they have received. While such guidance is helpful, it is the authors themselves who are to be congratulated for their enthusiasm, altruism, and ambition. They have brought together their collective and varied experiences in a series of monographs that will prove invaluable to any trainee with an impulse to ask a question, enquire more deeply, or challenge perceived wisdom.

The authors have set out the sequential processes of defining a research question, obtaining requisite permissions, collecting and analysing data, presenting results, and synthesising conclusions, all essential steps for those embarking on a research project. The importance of a detailed literature review and critical appraisal before embarking on a project is invaluable advice. Indeed, many would consider the words of an Irish proverb 'a good start is half the work' apply as readily to research as to any other endeavour.

Such complexities are not for the fainthearted. Collaboratives such as STARSurg offer medical students opportunities to become involved in an established project. As the authors attest, the opportunity to participate in a research project is often the stimulus to continue and to develop lifelong interest. For the busy clinician, regional, national, and international collaborative and multicentre clinical trails can answer research questions beyond the ability of individual units.

Scientific writing requires discipline and the ability to distil the subject matter to its essence. While social media provide boundless opportunities for collaboration, information exchange, and public engagement, peer review publication remains the benchmark. Remember one good paper in a prestigious journal is worth many lesser publications. Rejection is common and upsetting, but the reader should take heart. All of us have been there, thus the importance of resilience as set out in the last chapter.

For those embarking on a project, do not be afraid to start, and enjoy the satisfaction of answering the questions you have asked.

P. Ronan O'Connell, MD, FRCSI, FRCPS (Glas),
FRCS (Edin), FRCS (Eng), FCSHK
President Royal College of Surgeons in Ireland
Emeritus Professor of Surgery, University College Dublin

Preface

Over the last few decades, there has been a push towards evidence-based medicine, with the medical fraternity recognising and embracing the improved outcomes brought about by this approach. Central to this is the ability of healthcare professionals across all levels to be able to understand and undertake scientifically sound efforts to gather and learn from this evidence. This can be on a local level, for example, departmental audits, or on a national or international level, as is the case with large randomised controlled trials. Unfortunately, although academic medicine topics such as research and teaching are often discussed and taught at medical schools – many of which are at the forefront of international research efforts – medical students and junior doctors rarely get the chance to participate in any real-world studies, or indeed critique any practice changing studies in a meaningful way for themselves. The situation in regard to teaching is similar. Peer-to-peer teaching opportunities may be limited to self-arranged sessions with little to no guidance or formal training in how to do this key task, which will be crucial for the rest of one's career.

This is despite these activities being recognised as essential by undergraduate and postgraduate educators. In fact, they are a key part of selection for postgraduate employment. Candidates who demonstrate awareness of and proficiency with research and other academic activities such as teaching are highly sought after. However, many candidates, particularly those who don't take time out of their undergraduate programmes or pursue a higher degree, tend not to have had the exposure and opportunities to engage with these academic activities as students and junior healthcare professionals. Many will have never undertaken any formal research or teaching during this time. Furthermore, we have found that many students with an interest in medical research don't have the skills and experience required to get started, and they may lack mentors and senior colleagues with the time, interest, or experience to help them.

We were fortunate that, at an early stage in our training, either as students or junior doctors, we had access to high-quality research units with experienced mentors. This nurtured our interest, and we have since sought higher research degrees that have allowed us to explore this further. We have written this book for those who do not get this opportunity. This book is a guide to help at each step of the research process, providing personal examples to help you get started in medical research and to solve many of the challenges that you may encounter during this process.

This book will also be useful for any individual seeking to improve his or her knowledge and skills in medical research for personal use and for interview and examination preparation purposes. We have written this in a very practical manner, with real-life examples, with the hope that you will embrace the process and carry out meaningful research and teaching that is of interest to you and of benefit to the medical community.

Robert Foley
Robert Maweni
Shahram Shirazi
Hussein Jaafar

About the Companion Website

This book is accompanied by a website at:

www.wiley.com/go/foley/succeed

Scan the QR code:

The website includes:

- Gantt chart
- Sample consent form, Sample information leaflet, Sample proposal
- Sample posters and presentations

Chapter 1 **How to get involved in research**

1.1 Why do research?

Research involves logical and systematic investigation of a topic in order to reach new conclusions and to gain greater understanding. Research also fundamentally involves the recording of one's findings and the dissemination of the results to others, allowing for the research to be replicated. At its core, research is about finding the answer to meaningful questions. Research represents the backbone of progress within medicine. Becoming involved in research as a medical student, junior doctor, or healthcare professional is an incredibly valuable and rewarding tool to have in one's arsenal. The benefits offered by performing quality research are many; for example, research

- Demonstrates your interest in a topic.
- Allows you to build up your own knowledge base.
- Offers a stimulating reason to learn more about a topic.
- Can often keep you interested in your work.
- Allows you to become a better, more well-informed healthcare provider.
- May lead to improvements in your ability to provide patient care.
- Provides a great chance to improve your CV.

This book aims to offer a how to guide to starting your research career, whether you have any experience with research or not. Research involves time and effort. It is not always easy to start, continue, or to finish a project. However, if you are dedicated and invest your time wisely, you can succeed in medical research.

The goal of getting involved in research can be many of the above outlined benefits, but the main goal should be to gain experience in research, develop skills that will help you throughout your career, and decide how much of a research interest to pursue over the course of your career.

How to Succeed in Medical Research: A Practical Guide, First Edition.
Robert Foley, Robert Maweni, Shahram Shirazi, and Hussein Jaafar.
© 2021 John Wiley & Sons Ltd. Published 2021 by John Wiley & Sons Ltd.
Companion website: www.wiley.com/go/foley/succeed

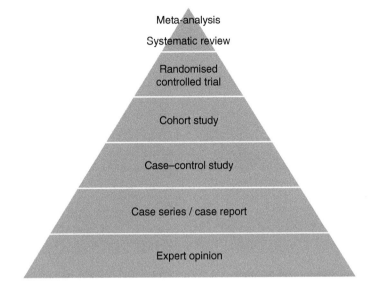

Figure 1.1 The hierarchy of evidence.

1.2 What can I become involved in?

There are a number of different areas of research within medicine. Broadly, there is pre-clinical research, which takes place in the laboratory, and clinical research, which takes place in a clinical setting such as a hospital. Clinical research will be the main focus of this book, and it is the easier branch to become involved in, especially if one is already working in the healthcare setting. We will also discuss pre-clinical research at various points throughout the course of the book.

Another important concept is the hierarchy of research (Figure 1.1). This hierarchy establishes what types of research publications are the most trustworthy and assigns each type a level of evidence. This is often represented as a pyramid and has evolved over the past few decades, guided by the principles of having the weakest study designs at the bottom and the most robust study designs at the top.

1.3 Different types of research

1.3.1 Case report

A case report involves the analysis of an interesting patient and the dissemination of the case and the interesting aspects of it to other healthcare professionals. It also generally involves a literature review to explain the context of the case in light of the current research on this topic. Although low down on the hierarchy of evidence, this is one of the best places to start if you are new to research. A case report allows you to perform many of the important parts of research, including discussion with colleagues, data collection, presentation, manuscript preparation, and submission for peer review. A more detailed guide of how to perform a case report is given in Chapter 9.

1.3.2 Case series
A case series is essentially the same as a case report except that it looks at more than one patient. The topic of the case series is generally one that means it is difficult to recruit large numbers of patients, and so the number in the series is usually small. This is also an excellent starting point for one's research journey and is discussed in Chapter 9.

1.3.3 Commentary
A commentary is a publication that offers the opinion of the authors on another newly published article. It usually will be offered by the editor of a journal to an expert on a particular topic. This may be difficult to become involved in; however, if you find a research mentor that is an expert in his or her field, it may be a potential opportunity to write a short but interesting piece.

1.3.4 Interesting approach
These articles are published in journals to highlight a technical skill or a new way of performing a common procedure. Because the focus is on a procedure, these are usually written by those who specialise in a surgical or interventional specialty. Again, this type of article will need heavy input from the senior colleague who performs the skill or technique, but it is a great opportunity to work in tandem with an expert and get started in research. Skills in manuscript preparation can be gained, and due to the technical nature of the article, it also offers the chance to develop skills in image editing/production for publication.

1.3.5 Letter
Ask senior colleagues if they have read a recent paper on which they have some opinions they would like to share or questions they would like to ask the author. In this way, you can become involved in writing a letter to the editor outlining these points. Letters can often be quite succinct and not take too much time to produce. However, often your mentor will not have the time to write a letter despite having excellent opinions and points on the topic. It is also a good chance for you to practice your writing and literature review.

Case Study 1.1 Letter to the editor [1]

One of my earliest mentors in research once commented that 'we should all be writing more letters to the editor'. Although it still happens, the concept is much less common than it was previously. It is an excellent opportunity to sum up one's thoughts on an article, to offer an alternative point of view, to ask any pressing questions of the authors, or to disagree with their conclusions. Often a letter to the editor and a reply from the original author can make for very interesting debate. While I was reading on the topic of quality of life in patients with a specific type of brain tumour (an acoustic neuroma), I came across a recently published paper by Lodder and colleagues [2]. I had written a similar paper previously and had read a number of similar papers in the preceding months. I was struck by how the paper and the conclusion focused on the same topic as everyone else. The authors found that patients with an acoustic neuroma had a similar quality of life outcome, whether they underwent treatment with surgery, radiotherapy, or both. However, the authors also found that overall, the quality of life scores were low in all patients. Unfortunately, this was not addressed in the article. Many papers with similar findings merely compared quality of life outcomes with different treatments rather than focus on the big picture – which is, that quality of life outcomes in these patients are low. It was my feeling that doctors should be aware that all patients with this disease may have a low quality of life, and so we must try to identify problems in every patient. It felt to me that many authors were ignoring the elephant in the room, and so I wrote to the editor to explain this point of view. Because it was something I felt strongly about, it was fun and relatively easy to write the letter.

1.3.6 Collaborative

Collaborative studies can be an excellent way to ease yourself into the research world. The main advantage is that it is simple! The lead authors will take care of most of the work, including the literature review, the research proposal, the ethical application, the data analysis, the write-up, and the submission process. The disadvantage is that in essence you can only be involved in the data collection. However, despite this obvious downside, it can still be quite a useful experience. The lead authors will provide lots of collaborators with a data collection plan, and you can follow this at your local institution. Usually, because collaborative studies use patients from lots of different areas, there is not too much data collection to be done, and so it may not take too much time. The reward can be gained without too much effort. The first thing to do is to find a collaborative study to become involved in. A number of different collaboratives exist, and there are often a number of options out there. For example:

- STARSurg – A student-led research collaborative with the aim to carry out large and impactful studies within surgery.
- BURST – A urology collaborative that will be discussed in the following case study.
- GlobalSurg – A research collaborative that aims to improve surgical outcomes through research on a global scale.

Case Study 1.2 MIMIC collaborative study [3]

I received an email advert for a new collaborative study being undertaken in the UK, called the MIMIC study, run by the BURST collaborative. The study was looking at patients presenting to the emergency department with renal colic (pain secondary to a kidney stone). I emailed the study lead to register my interest in collecting data on 50 patients at my local hospital. I also found one of the urology consultants at my hospital to ask if he would be interested in being the supervisor for this project. I then applied for ethical approval in my hospital, using the ethical application letter provided for me by the lead author.

Once this was approved by the ethics department, I was given an Excel file by the lead authors, with a number of pieces of information to collect on each of the 50 patients. Doing this took some time, including figuring out which IT systems to use. The MIMIC study involved 71 hospitals worldwide. The study was a great success, led to a number of presentations at national and international conferences, and received a number of prizes as well. The presentations were shared among the collaborators so that a number of people had the opportunity to present. I presented the findings of the study to my local hospital's urology department. The findings were also published in the *British Journal of Urology*, with all of the collaborators named. Although I took a peripheral role, the study was a worthwhile endeavour and a good chance to gain experience in research without having to do it all alone!

One alternative to becoming involved in a collaborative research project is to lead your own collaborative study. It is without doubt more work to do so, so I would recommend becoming involved as a collaborator first. However, the rewards can be immense, and if you have the time and the motivation, leading a collaborative is a great experience.

As you can see, the creation of a collaborative project gives the opportunity to engage in a multi-institutional project with a large number of clinical and research teams, to prepare and present research proposals, to complete

Case Study 1.3 Prostate cancer research collaborative

During some dedicated research time, I had the opportunity to lead a nationwide study throughout Ireland that sought to collect information on men undergoing prostate biopsy and to create an Irish prostate cancer risk assessment tool. Under the guidance of my MSc supervisor, I met with each of the department leads in urology at all eight tertiary urology centres operating under the National Cancer Control Programme in Ireland. I presented a research proposal to the heads of department, seeking to recruit patients for the study from each centre. I then completed the ethical review board applications for each hospital and recruited members to assist with the data collection. The number of patients recruited to this study was more than 4000. My role also included working on the statistical analysis of the data and enlisting the help of the biostatistics department at my university. The next step was the dissemination of the research findings and presentations at local, national, and international meetings. The project has led to a number of publications, and the research project has continued with patient recruitment and the development of more refined risk models, an ongoing interest in my research team.

ethical review board applications, to collect large numbers of data, to analyse and interpret the results with the appropriate statistical methodology, and to disseminate the findings. Although it may seem like a daunting task, it is incredibly rewarding, and throughout the sections in this text, we will discuss each of these stages and how to do it for yourself.

Collaboratives don't need to be big, formal organisations with national or international interests, as previously described. And, while large collaboratives are a great way to get started in research, or indeed, get your name on a publication, the topic of research chosen by collaborative leads may not be of particular interest to you, and being listed along with a very long list of co-authors may not appeal to you.

Therefore, it may be best to form what we term a 'pseudo-collaborative'. This is a small group of individuals who may share the same interest in a topic as you but are at other geographical locales and have different key skills and knowledge to bring to a research project.

Case Study 1.4 Learning outcomes in surgery collaborative [4]

I decided to pursue my interest in the teaching of surgical skills to Foundation Year 1 (FY1) doctors. This was important to me because this was the level at which I was working, and I was keen to find the best and easiest way to acquire surgical skills to help me on the way to becoming an ENT surgeon. I discussed this with my mentor, a foundation training programme director who was also a surgical consultant, and we came up with a curriculum of work-based assessments that, we felt, would prepare FY1 doctors for surgical training as well as allow them to enjoy their surgical FY rotations.

With the idea formed, it was important to recruit team members with expertise and reach that I lacked. I created a PowerPoint presentation with the idea and pitched it to colleagues at my level with greater statistics and recruitment expertise than I, as well as my former professor of surgery, all of whom I found to be receptive. The paper was later published, with data from across the UK and Ireland, which would not have been possible if working without collaboration.

1.3.7 Case–control study and cohort study

Original research is arguably the most important type of research to perform and should be the goal. The first step in original research will be to identify an interesting clinical question and then design a study to attempt to answer the question. For example, if we consider migraine-type headache, we could ask: what is the relationship between patients' migraine headache and patient clinical features? Are there any risk factors that predispose patients to migraine headache, such as age or weight? We can then look at a group of patients with migraine and a group of patients without migraine and compare the findings in both groups. This would be termed a 'case–control study'. These sorts of studies are retrospective in design and look back at risk factors in patients with a defined outcome (i.e. a diagnosis of migraine headache or not). Case–control studies can be an excellent starting point for original research because they are cheap and easy to perform.

In contrast to this, cohort studies look at a population of patients and compare those who were exposed to something and those that were not and then see what the outcomes are in each group. A classic example of this type of research is the Framingham Heart Study [5], which began in the 1940s. This study followed large numbers of patients from the beginning of the study and waited to see which patients developed heart disease. The researchers then looked back at the clinical features that differed between those patients who developed heart disease and those patients who did not. This study found correlations between heart disease and risk factors such as smoking, high cholesterol, and high blood pressure. The disadvantage of this type of study is that it requires large amounts of funding and takes a long time to conduct. Therefore, although this type of research can be very valuable, it is not the ideal place to start.

1.3.8 Randomised controlled trial

A randomised controlled trial (or RCT) is a very important study design utilised in medical research. It involves recruiting a cohort and randomly assigning the patients in the study to receive one treatment or another. In a double-blind trial design, the patients and the researchers also don't know which treatment the patient has been assigned. These trials are the best method of determining the optimal treatment strategy for patients in medicine. This method is commonly used in oncology for comparing new cancer treatments to the current gold standard treatment.

1.3.9 Systematic review and meta-analysis

This type of research involves summarising all of the research that has already taken place on a particular topic. There is a very detailed methodology to follow in conducting this sort of research, and the meta-analysis is also carried out in a particular fashion. This type of research can be very time-consuming when performed for the first time, but it can be an excellent way to gain an in-depth understanding of a topic and can also be very useful if you cannot identify a research question for a piece of original research.

1.4 Clinical vs laboratory

There is an important distinction between clinical and laboratory research. Clinical is undoubtedly easier to perform if you are new to research. Laboratory research is usually undertaken as part of a research degree, or sometimes an extended period of time is allocated to a research project in medical or biomedical degrees. Laboratory research takes time and can rarely be properly performed on a part-time basis while attempting to continue your regular studies or work. Laboratory research is discussed in more detail in Chapter 10.

1.5 Getting ideas for research

The ideas needed for research will depend on the type of research you plan to perform. For example, ideas for a case report or a case series may arise from time spent meeting patients in clinic or on the wards. Ideas may come from discussing your interest in getting involved in research with a senior colleague (more in Chapter 2), or you may not need to come up with the idea at all, such as in the case of a collaborative project.

Ask yourself: what interests or excites me in research? This is one of the main things to bear in mind when thinking of ideas for your research. It can be difficult to stay motivated in research at times; however, if you pick a topic that you have genuine interest in, it will be far easier to continue with the project until the end. Another excellent way to get ideas for research is to draw on the experience of your seniors. Try to identify those people who have been involved in research in the past and discuss it with them. What led them to become involved in research? How did they start? Who did they talk to? This kind of discussion can be very important, and if your senior is receptive, then you can use this person as a role model/mentor over the course of your research career.

Case Study 1.5 Identifying areas for research

I had the idea for a research study in patients with acoustic neuroma (a brain tumour) because a family member of mine was diagnosed with the condition. I obviously had a big interest in this disease, and I was particularly interested if patients with this tumour experienced a big impact on their quality of life. I discussed the idea with a colleague of mine, and this project was also perfect for him, as it allowed him to demonstrate his interest in ear, nose, and throat surgery, because that is who commonly looks after patients with acoustic neuroma. But we didn't know much about quality of life in research, so we asked for help from our hospital's psychiatric team, particularly concerning how to perform a quality of life assessment, and they gave us ideas of questionnaires we could use. From there, we spent some time reviewing the literature on the topic. We found that some research had been conducted on the topic, but that we could approach it from a different angle. We were interested in whether the quality of life was different in patients who had undergone a different treatment strategy, and if alcohol was used as a coping mechanism. We thought that our question was clinically interesting, and we decided that we would proceed to the next step in this study and try to identify a supervisor for the project.

References

1. Foley, R.W. (2019). Acoustic neuroma quality of life: are we missing the point? *Eur. Arch Otorhinolaryngol.* **276**: 1549–1550. https://www.ncbi.nlm.nih.gov/pubmed/29948270.
2. Lodder, W.L., van der Laan, B.F.A.M., Lesser, T.H., and Leong, S.C. (2018). The impact of acoustic neuroma on long-term quality-of-life outcomes in the United Kingdom. *Eur. Arch Otorhinolaryngol.* **275**: 709–717. https://www.ncbi.nlm.nih.gov/pubmed/29330600.
3. BURST Urology (2020). MIMIC study overview. https://bursturology.com/mimic (accessed 28 October 2020).

4. Maweni, R.M., Foley, R.W., Lupi, M. et al. (2016). Surgical learning activities for house officers: do they improve the surgical experience? *Ir. J. Med. Sci.* **185**: 913–919. https://www.ncbi.nlm.nih.gov/pubmed/27585806.
5. Framingham Heart Study (2020). Three generations of research on heart disease. https://www.framinghamheartstudy.org (accessed 28 October 2020).

Chapter 2 **Conducting a study**

2.1 How to find a research project

We have discussed in the previous chapter how to think of ideas for research projects. If you are lucky enough to have an idea, you can proceed to finding a mentor/supervisor for the project. However, if you have no idea where to start, then you will need to find a research project. One way to do this is to find an appropriate mentor/supervisor.

2.1.1 Use your interests

Again, an important factor is to ensure you think about projects in an area in which you have a particular interest. If you are interested in cardiology, find out who in your hospital or university has an active research interest in that area. Read through some of their previous publications to get an idea of the type of research they are engaging in. Although the papers may be quite detailed, they do give an overview of what the researchers are working with – e.g. perhaps they perform lots of clinical studies, perhaps they have a statistical focus, or perhaps they are performing lab experiments. Think about if this type of research will fit in with your plan.

2.1.2 Speak to your colleagues

Another helpful source of information is senior colleagues who have undertaken research projects in the past. Often you can find out who has done this through word of mouth, by looking at the posters in your department, or online. If you are in a university setting, look to your favourite lecturers or tutors for advice. Pick someone you think is a nice person and see if he or she can point you in the right direction. If the colleague performs research but not in the area that interests you, he or she can introduce you to the best person to talk to.

How to Succeed in Medical Research: A Practical Guide, First Edition.
Robert Foley, Robert Maweni, Shahram Shirazi, and Hussein Jaafar.
© 2021 John Wiley & Sons Ltd. Published 2021 by John Wiley & Sons Ltd.
Companion website: www.wiley.com/go/foley/succeed

2.1.3 Meeting your potential mentor

Once you have found someone you think could be your mentor, you need to arrange to meet the person. Find an email address online or by asking the secretary or some of the administrative staff. Email is an excellent way to first get in touch with someone, and it offers you the opportunity to think about what you would like to say, so you can put the best foot forward (see Case Study 2.1). When arranging a meeting, bring a pen and notepad with you to make any notes that you may forget. Make sure you have read some background information in your potential mentor's area of interest before the meeting. Try to leave the meeting with a plan for the next step, who you need to meet next, when you will next meet, what information you need to gather before the next meeting, and who else will need to be contacted. One of the keys to good research is being organised!

2.1.4 Research programmes

There are other great ways to find a project that can be less daunting. Many universities run research programmes, particularly with a focus on completing a short-term project over the summer period, whereas other programmes are built into certain degrees by default. Try to find out about research internships and student summer research programmes in your local area. These programmes are extremely valuable to the research teams because they can benefit from an extra pair of hands without having to hire another member of staff. Because of this, there are often several available positions to choose from.

Case Study 2.1 University college dublin student summer research

As a pre-clinical medical student, I was given the opportunity to complete a 10-week supervised research project in my university. I identified a topic that interested me from the list of available projects online and completed the application form. I then emailed the professor who was the lead researcher on the project. The following are the email and an excerpt from the application form.

Email:

***

Dear Prof.,

Please find attached my application form for the Student Summer Research Programme. I would be very grateful if you would consider me for the project this summer. I am currently in Medicine Stage 4 and I am available from June 24th until August 23rd. Ideally we could discuss what you would require of me and what the period of research would entail, just a chance for me to understand a bit more about the project. Please just let me know if and when this would be convenient and I'll make myself available.

Thank you for your time, I look forward to hearing from you.

***

Application Form:

***

Q: In 100 words maximum, give reasons why you should be selected to undertake this summer research project: Evaluation of Prostate Cancer Risk Prediction Tools.

A: I am keen to participate in this research programme to expand my knowledge, skills, and experience in the field of medical research; noting that research plays a significant role towards improving the quality of life of patients. I am particularly interested in this research because, to me, I believe this project can have a real impact on diagnostic strategies employed to assess patients with suspected prostate cancer. It seems to me that a need for this study exists, especially in this specific cancer, considering the variable expressivity of the disease. That is, some patients with prostate cancer, proven by a biopsy, may never show symptoms and die with the disease as opposed to from it. And so I feel that finding the most appropriate risk prediction tool is particularly important.

***

After an interview, I was selected for the position. The interview took the form of a casual discussion between myself and my supervisor, in which we got to know each other a bit better and I was given more of a detailed background to the research project. After the 10-week period, I presented a poster of my work at the Student Summer Research Awards. My mentor helped me create my first poster presentation and practiced with me before the big day. There was also a communication workshop organised for all of the students in the programme to prepare for the presentations. In this way, I was taken through the research process from the beginning of a project to the dissemination of the results.

2.1.5 Is this the right project for me?

One of the hardest parts of research is finding the right project. Often, we can be asked to do a project for someone in an informal way. However, it is incredibly important to learn which studies are worth your time and which are not. Learning how to say no can be difficult, but it is an essential skill to develop. If a project sounds fantastic, then by all means get involved. But if it doesn't sound like a useful project to you, think about it hard before committing your valuable time to something you don't think will work out. Think about the person or people offering the project to you; do they have a research background? Have they looked into whether this research has already been performed and already been published? Have they brought projects through to completion, leading to presentations and publications? These are the important questions to ask yourself before committing to a project, so make sure to do your 'research' on who you are getting involved with!

2.2 How to approach a mentor

Once you have found someone you think would make a good mentor, you will need to approach him or her. Sometimes the best approach is to send an email or to knock on the person's door and introduce yourself! Sometimes it can be hard to find a busy clinician in a hospital setting. You will need to do your research and figure out the best time and method to find and approach your mentor. The following case studies outline how to approach a mentor, both the easy way and the less easy way!

Case Study 2.2 The direct approach

While a medical student, I had developed an interest in radiology as a specialty, and I was keen to learn more about it. We had a particularly enthusiastic lecturer – he was a keen teacher and kept things light-hearted. I particularly enjoyed the way he displayed his images on screen and he kept his explanations simple and understandable. I had never undertaken any research, and I didn't know where to begin. I decided to approach him after a lecture and discuss. How I could learn a bit more, express an interest in radiology, and get started in research? We had a short chat, and I felt quite encouraged afterwards. I decided to send him a follow-up email the next week.

***

Dear Dr.,

I was speaking to you last Monday about an opportunity to spend some time in radiology undertaking some clinical research. I am very eager to find a research opportunity this summer and I'd love for it to be in an area of interest for me. I hope to confirm my interest in pursuing radiology and hopefully having research to my name in the area will stand to me in the future.

I've enjoyed your lectures this term, and I have taken an optional module in radiology and diagnostic imaging last semester, and I'd be very grateful if you can find a position for me this summer.

Thank you for your time, I look forward to hearing from you.

***

He got back to me quickly and arranged to meet me in his office at the hospital a couple of days later. He explained to me that at my stage it would be better to try and undertake some basic science research, as the clinical research could be done later in my training. He directed me towards a colleague of his at the university, and this was how I began my first steps in research. Although not what I was expecting and leading me far away from radiology, this meeting was incredibly beneficial and led me down the best route to begin my research career.

However, it is not always that simple. Sometimes you may need to be persistent, and the following case study demonstrates the value of persistence. You may need to think on your feet and explore other avenues of achieving your goals. You may need to convince a potential mentor that you are worth working with.

Case Study 2.3 The indirect approach

As previously mentioned in Chapter 1, I was interested in conducting a study in acoustic neuroma. There is only one neurosurgical centre in Ireland that deals with this condition, and it was not twinned with my university's hospital. Because of this, it was going to be less straightforward to get the study up and running.

I looked up the website of the hospital with a neurosurgical team and found the consultants who managed patients with acoustic neuroma. I found the lead consultant of the department and attempted to contact him by email. Unfortunately this was unsuccessful, and we received no response. I then decided to try and talk to his secretary. We had a phone discussion and the secretary kindly agreed to print my email as a letter and hand it to the consultant.

***

Dear Mr.,

Enclosed please find the research proposal for 'Self Reported Quality of Life and Psychosocial Outcomes in Vestibular Schwannoma Patients in Ireland'.

We propose to conduct a study of vestibular schwannoma patients in Ireland to ascertain the impact of this disease on patient quality of life and mental health. We hope to obtain patients for this study from your clinic and we would very much appreciate your help in this regard.

In terms of background information, I am a medical student and have completed five years of my undergraduate degree and have a keen interest in pursuing this piece of research.

We hope that you will allow us to conduct this study under your guidance. My contact details are outlined below, and I look forward to hearing from you.

Sincerely,

***

However, this was again an unsuccessful attempt, and we received no response. The next step was to find a way to meet him in person. I decided to visit the neurosurgery department in person and see if I could find some more information. I went to the outpatient department and found the nursing staff there, who directed me to the acoustic neuroma specialist nurse. I managed to find her office, and we had a great chat, where she explained the best times during the week to meet the elusive consultant. Every Monday morning at 8 a.m., he would begin a meeting before his acoustic neuroma clinic, where each patient would be discussed. I arranged to come on a Monday morning with my research colleague to discuss our proposal with him in person. I printed off our cover letter and proposal and put it inside a binder (to give a look of professionalism) and brought this with me. We entered the meeting conference room and introduced ourselves, presented him with our proposal, and asked if he would be our project supervisor. He was delighted with our efforts and happy to have us on board. Although it took a good deal of effort to eventually get his backing for the study, once we had met and discussed the project in person, the response was very favourable.

2.3 Planning your study

2.3.1 Defining a research question

The first step in a research project is deciding what to research. Often the idea for this may come from a mentor or a supervisor who has identified an interesting question over the course of his or her clinical practice. However, it is also possible to come up with interesting questions yourself. This is an especially important point, because if you choose a question that interests you personally, it will be much easier to maintain your interest in the research.

It is vital that you take plenty of time to decide on a research question. The first step is to pick a broad topic that you would like to research – for example, 'heart failure'. Once you have selected this, try to refine your idea so that you are focusing on a manageable area within your topic of interest. For instance, you may decide that you are interested in the efficacy of medications for heart failure. Now you can begin to formulate questions related to this topic, such as, What medications are the most effective in reducing symptoms of heart failure? How many patients taking a certain medication experience fewer symptoms of heart failure? These questions can also be framed in a laboratory research context: What is the effect of a certain medication on the immune cells of heart failure patients?

A common method of formulating a research question is the PICO method. This method involves thinking about the Patient, Intervention, Comparison, and Outcome in order to decide on a logical research question. For example, you may see a 74-year-old man in clinic with heart failure and the decision is made to start a new medication, digoxin, because the patient has been hospitalised with increasing frequency over the last three months. You are interested in whether or not digoxin will decrease the patient's risk of being admitted to hospital. In this scenario, the PICO method can be applied.

- Patient: 74-year-old man with heart failure.
- Intervention: Digoxin.
- Comparison: Best medical therapy without digoxin.
- Outcome: Rate of hospitalisation.

The research question then becomes, 'In elderly men with heart failure, is digoxin effective in reducing the need for hospitalisation?'

Case Study 2.4 Acoustic neuroma study

The PICO method can easily be applied to our acoustic neuroma research project, as previously discussed in Chapter 1.

• Patient: Acoustic neuroma patients.

• Intervention: Surgery.

• Comparison: Radiotherapy or conservative management.

• Outcome: Quality of life.

Our research question was: In patients with acoustic neuroma, does surgical management in comparison to radiotherapy and conservative treatment lead to different quality of life outcome?

Case Study 2.5 Prostate cancer biomarkers

When I joined the prostate cancer research team at my university, my supervisor was interested in how to better identify men with prostate cancer. The current gold standard blood test was called prostate-specific antigen (PSA). We were interested in whether or not a new blood test called the prostate health index (PHI) would perform better than PSA. Again, the PICO method can be used to formulate our research question:

• Patient: Men.

• Intervention: PHI blood test.

• Comparison: PSA blood test.

• Outcome: Diagnosis of prostate cancer.

In men, is the PHI test superior to PSA in the identification of prostate cancer? This question then became the foundation for the research to follow and is the question that our research aimed to answer.

2.3.2 Literature search and literature review

A thorough literature review is essential prior to beginning a research project. This achieves a number of different goals and will provide you with the latest evidence on your chosen research topic. This will set the scene for how much research has already been carried out on this topic and whether the research question has been answered yet. It is also a great practice to get into, as it will give you an excellent knowledge base from which to plan your study. How to carry out a literature review is covered in detail in Chapter 3.

2.3.3 Study design

When it comes to designing a study, it is important to know what type of research you wish to carry out. Do you wish to write up a case report? Or do you want to carry out an intervention and assess the participants' responses? Research design can be quantitative, relying on measurements made in numbers, or qualitative, which collects data that cannot be easily summarised with numbers, such as a patient's feelings about a particular medication he or she is taking. Within quantitative research, you can have different types of studies. For example, you may perform a questionnaire in your patient population to answer your research question or you may take patients who underwent a certain treatment and compare those patients who responded well and those who did not.

Within medicine, certainly when beginning your career in research, we recommend focusing on a quantitative project. We would also recommend attempting an observational study, as there will not be a need for an intervention. This is in contrast to an experimental study, in which a new intervention is undertaken and the response is assessed. In an observational study, you are interested in describing what is occurring in a particular topic or in the relationship between different things.

The study design you select will depend on your research question. For example, my research question may be: In patients presenting to the emergency department with acute abdominal pain, what is the rate of appendicitis? I can answer this question using an observation study design, in which I gather data on patients presenting to the emergency department and finding out what diagnosis was made. In another example, my research question may be: In patients presenting to the emergency department with acute abdominal pain, what is the relationship between the patient's temperature and the diagnosis of appendicitis? This question can be answered with an observational study, which gathers data on patients presenting to the emergency department, each patient's temperature, and the final diagnosis.

2.3.4 Analysis plan

Once you have decided on a study design, the next step is the creation of an analysis plan. This is a key component of your research study, and it is important to plan this correctly so that your analysis can be done simply once all the data is collected. You will need to think of the important pieces of information you want to collect to answer your research question. In the example just mentioned, regarding acute appendicitis, the key information to collect is as follows:

- Number of patients presenting to the emergency department with acute abdominal pain in a certain time period (e.g. 3 months).
- Temperature of each patient.
- Final diagnosis, i.e. did the patient have appendicitis or an alternative diagnosis?

If you collect these three pieces of information, you can answer the research question you have posed. It is important to think of what type of information you are collecting as well. Is it a yes/no piece of information, a categorical variable, such as diagnosis of appendicitis or not? Or is it a piece of information that could be a wide range of values, a continuous variable, such as temperature? This is important because it will impact what type of statistical analysis you will perform on these variables. We will discuss statistical analysis in more detail in Chapter 5, which will help you to create your analysis plan. A sample analysis plan is shown in the next case study.

Case Study 2.6 Analysis plan

In a prostate cancer study we were performing, we were interested in the use of a blood test called PSA in the diagnosis of prostate cancer. We wanted to find out whether the levels of PSA differed between patients with prostate cancer and those without. We also wanted to know how effective this blood test was at differentiating between these two groups of patients – in other words, how good is PSA in the diagnosis of prostate cancer.

The key information to collect in this case is:

• Patients who have had a PSA level.

• The final diagnosis in each patient, i.e. prostate cancer or an alternative.

Firstly, we wanted to see the difference between PSA levels in patients with cancer and those without. PSA is a blood test that can have a wide range of numerical values; for example, one patient may have a PSA level of 0.1 while another can have a level of 100. This is therefore a continuous variable. We want to compare this continuous variable in two groups, and this can be done by comparing the average level in each group, otherwise known as the mean. These values can be compared using the t-test. Next, create a table such as the one below, which outlines the analysis to take place. In this way, once your data is collected, it is clear how the analysis will occur.

	Group 1 (patients with cancer)	Group 2 (patients without cancer)	Statistical test
PSA level			t-test

Using this example, and Chapter 5 on 'Analysing Your Data', you will be able to create your own analysis plan for your research study prior to beginning the data collection process.

2.3.5 Sample size

Estimating the number of patients you will need to answer your research question is an important step you must take before you begin your study. This is called 'sample size estimation'. It will inform you of how many patients to include in your study and how much data to collect. Estimating the required sample size can be complex, but in essence it depends on the main question you wish to answer – the primary outcome measure of your study. This will change depending on whether you are examining a continuous variable or a categorical variable. The type of analysis you can carry out on your data is discussed in more detail in Chapter 5. Sample size calculators are available online or within the statistical programme of your choice, but before using one, there are some concepts to understand.

The sample size estimation requires the researcher to define the type 1 (alpha) error and power. These are usually set at standard values of 0.05 for alpha error and 0.80 for power. These terms relate to the relationship of reality and the hypothesis of the study. For example, a study is conducted to analyse the relationship between smoking and lung cancer. The hypothesis is that there is a relationship between smoking and the incidence of lung cancer in a cohort of patients. The reality could be that there is a relationship or not, and the results of our study could show a relationship or no relationship. This is summarised in Table 2.1.

The alpha error is the probability of incorrectly rejecting our hypothesis – in other words, the chance that in reality there is a relationship and our study demonstrates that there is no relationship. In sample size estimation this would be a bad outcome, and so we set this value quite low and only accept the risk of that happening at 5%, or an alpha error of 0.05. The beta error is the chance that the hypothesis is wrongly accepted, whereas the opposite of this is power. Power is the probability that the incorrect hypothesis is correctly rejected, and our study will demonstrate the hypothesis to be false. The power value is generally set at 80%, or 0.8.

Table 2.1 Hypothesis testing.

	Reality relationship	Reality no relationship
Study shows a relationship	The hypothesis is accepted	The hypothesis is wrongly accepted *Beta error*
Study shows no relationship	The hypothesis is wrongly rejected *Alpha error*	The hypothesis is correctly rejected *POWER (1 – Beta)*

Once you have an analysis plan, with the research question you wish to answer and method of analysis you will be using, you can then calculate the required sample size.

Case Study 2.7 Surgical learning activities

In a paper we have published, we were interested in analysing the satisfaction of junior doctors who were working in a surgical specialty in the hospital. Each student was to undertake a 3- or 4-month job in surgery, and then we would assess his or her satisfaction with the job by questionnaire. There would then be two groups, those dissatisfied and those satisfied. We estimated that 30% of the dissatisfied participants would achieve their learning objectives, while we estimated that 60% would achieve them in the satisfied group. We also estimated that twice as many participants would be from the satisfied group, as these people were more likely to take the time to fill in our questionnaire. This allowed us to calculate the sample size as follows: Sample size calculation to compare two proportions was performed with a 5% probability of a type 1 error (alpha), 80% power, and an estimated average incidence of completed learning events of 60% and 30% in groups satisfied and dissatisfied with their surgical rotation. A ratio of respondents of 1:2 for those satisfied with surgical experience provided a minimum sample size of 95 to detect a statistically significant difference.

2.3.6 How to write a research proposal

A research proposal should outline the main objectives of your study, while also summarising the main research that has already been conducted on the topic, why this research question is of interest, and how you plan to go about conducting the study.

The main headings that can be included are as follows:

- Introduction.
- Background and Significance.
- Aim/Objectives/Purpose of Study.
- Methods.
- Hypothesis.
- Conclusion and Justification.

Essentially the research proposal will act as an excellent starting point for your research. If you have a research idea but do not yet have a supervisor, the proposal can allow you to organise your thoughts and can be used as a discussion point in a meeting. You can send your proposal in an email or bring it with you when you meet with a potential supervisor. If you already have a mentor/supervisor, then the proposal is still essential, as you will need it when applying for ethical approval. To write an effective proposal, you will need to conduct a thorough literature review, and this is discussed in Chapter 3. Please see the online content for a sample research proposal.

2.3.7 Ethical approval

Once the proposal is finished, in many cases you will need ethical approval. Completing and submitting the ethical application is the final step prior to data collection and will be a far less daunting task when you have completed the above steps in this chapter. Ethical approval is needed for research studies; however, in many regions ethical approval is not required if your study is considered a service evaluation project or clinical audit. In the UK, this is governed by the Medical Research Council and Health Research Authority, and it may differ worldwide. Check with your local research/ethics department and with your supervisor to find out what type of approval you need to apply for. Medical ethics and ethical approval is covered in more detail in Chapter 4.

2.3.8 Other considerations

2.3.8.1 Timelines

It is incredibly important to think about how long each portion of your research journey is going to take. As you can see from this chapter, there are a number of things to tackle before you can begin your data collection. And as you can probably imagine, these things take time to complete, especially if you are also working a full-time job or in full-time study. Try to plan out the timeline of your research journey as much as possible so that you can have a realistic plan of action.

An excellent way of planning out your time is through the use of a Gantt chart. This is essentially a to-do list with a timeline. It takes the form of a diagram that breaks down your project into smaller chunks and demonstrates how long you think each chunk will take. Then as you progress through your project, you can adjust and edit the chart to show your progress. Not only will this be a fantastic start to a project and facilitate your discussions with your supervisor, it is also an excellent way to keep track of your progress. There is a sample Gantt chart provided for you in the online content that comes with this book.

2.3.8.2 Motivation

When carrying out a research project, it is important that you are the driving force behind the project! As mentioned earlier, pick a topic you are interested in and you think will help you stay motivated for the lifespan of the project. Research can take years to complete, and often much research is left uncompleted for a variety of reasons. If you want your research to be successful, it will rarely be handed to you and made easy for you; YOU MUST BE THE DRIVING FORCE!

2.3.8.3 Speak to the previous researcher

Often, your research project will build upon the work of someone else. If possible, find that person and speak to him or her. Other researchers will be a great source of information that can really help your project to get up and running. They can also give you a great idea of a realistic timeline, while also alerting you to the pitfalls you may encounter. Ask if they are interested in keeping in touch and staying involved with your project. They may be extremely helpful if you encounter problems or get stuck, and they will no doubt be able to add value when it comes to presenting your work at conferences, writing your paper, and submitting for peer review.

2.3.8.4 Grant applications

If available, grants can provide income to help you to carry out your project. Although grant applications, in general, are for large-scale research and can offer huge sums of money, there are also smaller grants out there for smaller research projects. Keep your eyes and ears open to any possibilities that may be suitable for your research.

Case Study 2.8 Grant application

As discussed in Case Study 1.4, we carried out a study into the surgical learning activities carried out by junior doctors across the UK and Ireland. From this research we found that providing junior doctors with a list of important learning objectives allowed them to achieve more and to have a better experience in the workplace. We decided, therefore, that we should carry out a further study, in which we randomise junior doctors to either receive or not receive this checklist. Our hypothesis was that junior doctors receiving the checklist would benefit from this intervention. If proved correct, we would then recommend the checklist be rolled out across the UK and Ireland for all junior doctors, and we would have robust evidence to support this.

As luck would have it, the Association of Surgeons in Training had put out a call for grant applications. The grant was for £500 to support a surgical research project and required a research proposal, letter of support from the research supervisor, and the applicant's CV. We had already written our research proposal, and we could refer to our previous work and demonstrate that our research question was a valid one. We submitted our application and were awarded the grant to support our research. This allowed us to set up a website to carry out the study, with the study participants able to log their learning experiences online.

2.4 Data collection

Potentially the most important aspect of a research study is to clearly delineate your research question, design your study, and think about what problems may be encountered prior to beginning data collection. Once you have planned your study and completed the above steps in this chapter, the next step is to plan your data collection.

2.4.1 Plan

It is important to have a well-defined plan on what information you are going to collect. Make a spreadsheet that includes all of the data you will need to collect and discuss this with your supervisor prior to beginning data collection. There is nothing worse than having to go back and get one piece of data on everyone in your study. Some of the data to collect will be very obvious. You will know from your analysis plan what the main variables to collect are, because these are the ones that will answer your research question. However, during your literature review, you will likely notice that there is much more to it than that. There are many basic clinical pieces of information that you will need to also collect. These include basic information such as patient age and sex. This allows the reader to better understand the population you are studying. To return to an earlier example: if we are interested in the relationship between each patient's temperature and whether each was diagnosed with acute appendicitis, we may also collect information on the patient's age, sex, heart rate, blood pressure, and blood test results. Make sure you know exactly what to collect before you begin.

2.4.2 Where is the data?

This is another important piece of the puzzle. In some hospitals or other healthcare settings, you may need to collect data from paper notes, in which case you will need to request access to the patient's files from the medical records department. Often patient information is stored in electronic records, and sometimes you will need to access a number of different software systems on the hospital computers to find what you need. This will also require you, as the researcher, to have access to these systems, and you may need to discuss this with the IT department before beginning data collection.

2.4.3 Practical aspects

Another issue is where you will be able to collect the data. Is there a room in the department you work in that you can use to look through paper notes? Is there a free computer you can use to access electronic records? What time of the day will you be allowed to use this space for data collection?

2.4.4 Time

As you can imagine, all of these steps take time. But often, data collection can take a lot of time as well. You will need to plan carefully how you can dedicate the required time to collect all of the data. If the task seems overwhelming, you may need to recruit help with the collection process. However, if you do so, you will need to train the new data collector(s) effectively so that the data will be collected correctly and the results of your study will be as accurate as possible.

2.4.5 Storage and safety

To ensure that patient confidentiality is maintained, you will need to think about how the data is stored, in what fashion it is stored, and how you maintain the safety of this data. The principle of data collection in medical research is to minimise the amount of patient identifiable information that you collect and to minimise the number of people who have access to this data. This is any information that may allow someone to identify who the information refers to. The most obvious of these is the patient's name; however, date of birth or the patient's hospital number are also identifiable.

Any information collected that is identifiable must be stored safely. If on paper, this information should be kept in a locked drawer, in a locked room, preferably that of your supervisor to ensure its safety. This would apply to patient questionnaires. Identifiable data stored on a computer should be stored on the hospital or university system and be password protected. If this data is shared, it should be done so in an anonymised fashion or a pseudo-anonymised fashion. Anonymised data will remove all identifiable data, while pseudo-anonymised data will assign each patient with a new unique ID number. Then the data is non-identifiable unless you have the original data with the patient's information and unique ID. This allows you to share the data with other researchers in your team, but you can also make sure the data has been analysed correctly by referring back to the original data if needed.

Even if the data has been anonymised or pseudo-anonymised, if taking off the hospital computer or shared in electronic form, this data should be sent via a secure email only or shared via an encrypted USB. Often your IT department at your hospital or university will be able to provide an encrypted USB and a secure email service. The Medical Research Council (http://mrc.ukri.org) provides further detailed information on the use of patient information in research.

Chapter 3 **Literature review and critical appraisal**

Literature review and critical appraisal are part of a single, continuous process. It is important to perform a good critical appraisal of the articles you unearth during your literature review. The information garnered from this process is useful in planning your study, as discussed in the last chapter, as well as when writing and presenting the results of your study, which will be discussed in more detail later in the book. More than this, however, being able to critically appraise research will be a very useful skill in your work as a healthcare professional. This skill will allow you to make the best decisions for patient care and to appraise research for your department's or hospital's journal club. The ability to perform a literature review and present your findings in a logical and articulate manner will earn you numerous brownie points with your seniors.

3.1 Literature review

A literature review provides an insight into relevant current knowledge on a particular topic. As previously mentioned, the information gathered in this section may be useful for planning your study – providing you with comparable studies and information of the current state of play within your topic of interest. It is also incredibly useful for writing the introduction and discussion sections of your paper, in which case you will be looking to set out where in the realms of that topic of interest your study fits. Indeed, the highest component of the hierarchy of evidence, a systematic review, is at its core, an organised and logical literature review of published studies to answer a specific question. We, therefore, advocate undertaking literature reviews in a systematic and thorough manner to ensure you have a broad understanding of the topic and the evidence available.

How to Succeed in Medical Research: A Practical Guide, First Edition.
Robert Foley, Robert Maweni, Shahram Shirazi, and Hussein Jaafar.
© 2021 John Wiley & Sons Ltd. Published 2021 by John Wiley & Sons Ltd.
Companion website: www.wiley.com/go/foley/succeed

There are a number of tools that can help with various elements of this process, for example, Zotero and Mendeley. These free software programmes allow you to organise your research as well as cite and create bibliographies in a user-friendly way. We particularly like Zotero because it allows us to make notes on each article as we read it as well as pull various elements into our review document and cite the documents in whichever style we prefer – usually Vancouver, with a reliable and accurate bibliography. You should also have a word processing software with which you are comfortable, for example, Microsoft Word or the freely available Google Docs.

One method for performing a literature review is to have a split screen on your device, with the article you are reading on one side and the other side of the screen displaying the notes you are taking on each article as you read through it. We advise breaking down your notes document into sections. Place a 'Background' section at the top of your notes and a 'Discussion' section below, making notes into the appropriate section as you read. For example, epidemiological information can be entered under the 'Background' section and important results that can be used to draw comparison with your own study are placed in the 'Discussion' section. This will make writing the 'Introduction' and 'Discussion' sections of your paper much easier later on.

3.2 Search terms

Once you have decided on your topic of interest and defined your question using the PICO method, it is important to decide on your search terms. This is the list of words you will use to search through the database of medical literature, attempting to find all of the relevant studies that have previously been published.

Case Study 3.1 Medical electives study

This study examines a relatively niche aspect of medical education, thus defining search terms that would identify all of the useful and relevant literature was a challenge. We, therefore, took the approach of gathering as much of the literature as was available and then performing quick reviews of each article to decide whether or not it was relevant. The irrelevant articles were discarded, while the useful ones were kept for closer review. This is something that becomes easier with experience, but using a software program like Zotero makes the process much quicker.

We initially used the broad term 'medical elective', and then the synonymous 'medical clerkship' and 'foreign elective'. Similarly, one might use 'cancer' and then the synonymous 'malignancy'. As our study was looking at the safety implications for medical students and patients related to medical electives as well as the curriculum attached to medical electives, we added the search terms 'curriculum', 'ethics', 'patient', 'safety', and 'objectives' to our search term list.

3.2.1 Tips for search terms

An initial search may also help you to identify other useful terms; for example, on an initial literature search for articles discussing 'laryngopyocoele', it became apparent that another name for this is 'pyolaryngocoele'. Adding this new word to the list of search terms unlocked a significant number of articles.

There are situations where it may be useful to look at spelling variants, particularly taking care to use both American and British spellings of words such as 'oesophagus' (British English) and 'esophagus' (American English).

Furthermore, the medical fraternity is known to like using abbreviations, particularly TLAs (three-letter acronyms). It is, therefore, advisable to make sure to search for the most commonly used acronyms that relate to your topic. For example, in a study looking at knee injuries, it would be important to also search for 'ACL' (anterior collateral ligament) or 'PCL' (posterior collateral injury).

3.3 Where to search

Once you have decided on your search terms, it's time to search a database. For medical research, the first database we recommend searching is PubMed. PubMed includes the MEDLINE database, which is the United States' database of biomedical and life sciences and thus contains access to thousands of pertinent journals. It also has a simple, user-friendly interface, consisting of a simple search box. Other useful search engines include the Cochrane Library, Science Direct, and Google Scholar, though most of the articles you find there will also be found on PubMed.

There are other databases you can search, such as EMBASE, Web of Sciences, PsycINFO, and CINAHL, though some of them are not specific to health, biomedical, and life sciences. Your institute may also have its own search engine/library, which, once you have logged in, not only finds articles for you but also gives you access to them. For example, the UK National Health Service's Healthcare Databases Advanced Search (https://hdas.nice.org.uk) gives immediate access to articles and searches multiple databases once you are logged in. Access to this service is through the hospital library, and the ability to access articles all in one location is highly advantageous, as otherwise it can take significant amounts of time trying to get access to the articles via each journal website.

A benefit of PubMed is that it gives you access to free articles, and where the articles are not free, it provides you with links to where you can download the article, either via paying for it or through institutional access. We recommend taking advantage of your university or hospital's institutional access, and where you are not aware how to do this, your local librarian can show you how. Librarians are also helpful where your institution does not have access to an article, as they will look to acquire it via an inter-library loan.

3.4 How to search

The simplest way to search for articles of interest is to enter the keywords you have listed into your databases of choice. You will, however, often find an 'advanced' section where you can use your keywords with the Boolean operators AND, OR, and NOT to narrow or broaden your search as appropriate.

In our medical electives article, we were able to significantly narrow down the search with these operators. An example of a search we used was 'medical electives' AND 'ethics' AND 'safety', which allowed us to find the few articles that specifically dealt with this aspect of medical electives. The NOT operator will help you narrow articles down by excluding articles with any terms that you don't want to return.

3.5 Critical appraisal

Once you have performed your search and identified relevant articles, you should carry out critical appraisal of the articles. At its most basic level, critical appraisal is the process of assessing the strengths and weaknesses of a study, particularly how it was conducted and, therefore, the validity and applicability of the results. This is important because not all studies are created equal – there is a hierarchy of evidence, as discussed in Chapter 1. Furthermore, even in studies at the same level of hierarchy, they may differ in design such that they have varying strengths and weaknesses. In order to understand these strengths and weaknesses, it is important to be aware of a number of terms, and to consider the article in light of these.

3.5.1 Bias

The robustness of a study design is determined by its likelihood of introducing bias. Bias is best thought of as a systematic error, inherent to the study design, which can lead to the wrong conclusions. There are multiple types and we will discuss some of the most commonly encountered sources of bias.

3.5.1.1 Selection bias

This occurs where there is a selection of study participants without randomisation. This can be, either by the researcher or self-selection by participants who volunteer into a study. This introduces error by uneven comparison – potentially including certain confounders, which may have had an impact on the result.

3.5.1.2 Performance bias

This occurs where study participants and/or those undertaking the study are not blinded. Participants who know they are receiving an intervention are more likely to have a placebo effect, whilst researchers who are giving the intervention are more likely to act preferentially to those whom they know are receiving an intervention under investigation.

3.5.1.3 Recall bias
This occurs where some study participants are more or less likely to remember certain experiences than other participants. It is more likely in studies where participants are asked to self-report.

3.5.1.4 Attrition bias
This is found in trials where participants have been excluded or, somehow lost to follow up, such that their outcomes are not part of the final data set, therefore making it incomplete. This could occur for example in a study of an educational course with participants filling in a pre-course and post-course questionnaire. If some participants had performed the pre-course questionnaire but not the post-course questionnaire, there would be an attrition bias.

3.5.1.5 Reporting bias
This kind of bias can be found in any study where there is potential for selective reporting, and therefore, compromise of the results. For example, we conducted a study in which patients filled in a quality of life questionnaire. This study was subject to potential reporting bias, as patients who have a particularly good or bad outcome may feel more strongly about filling in the questionnaire. Any study that uses a questionnaire design, and relies on participants to choose whether or not to complete the questions is subject to this type of bias.

3.5.1.6 Nonresponse bias
Also known as participation bias, this type of bias occurs in a situation when the researcher cannot know the results that would have been attained, if those who did not participate or respond, actually participated. This is a very common cause of bias in studies, which invite people to participate, such as a questionnaire study. This type of bias can also occur secondary to attrition bias.

3.5.2 Confounding factors
These are factors which could, plausibly, explain the results of a study. They are, somehow, linked to the outcome of interest. One can often intuitively identify them e.g. in our Surgical Learning Activities study, in which we hypothesised that a curriculum of Work Based Assessments would lead to increased job satisfaction for Foundation Year 1 doctors. In this situation, confounders are other factors which could also lead to improved job satisfaction,

such as surgical subspecialty assignment and geographical location. It is not always obvious; however, therefore it is important to perform a comprehensive literature review to see what other writers in the field have done, as well as to discuss with your supervisor and research team as part of the planning phase.

3.5.3 Validity

Validity is a further measure of the quality of a study and is considered under the headings of 'Internal Validity' and 'External Validity'.

3.5.3.1 Internal validity

Internal validity refers to how well the study has prevented the systematic errors of bias and confounding in its design. It refers to the inherent reliability of the study.

3.5.3.2 External validity

External validity refers to how well the study results can be applied to the population of interest. It is a measure of how generalisable the study results are to a real-world scenario.

3.5.4 Models of critical appraisal

When appraising a study, it is helpful to have an objective and structured method. Over the years a number of these have been created, including scales (e.g. Jadad scale), domains (e.g. Cochrane risk of bias tool), and checklists (e.g. the Critical Appraisal Skills Programme [CASP] checklist). We will focus on CASP because we have found it to be the most user friendly and a commonly used method of appraising a study.

The CASP team has developed a variety of appraisal checklists, each specifically suited for a particular study, including systematic reviews, randomised controlled trials, case control studies, and cohort studies. These are available on their website (http://www.casp-uk.net) with print and electronic versions available, which one simply needs to fill with information regarding the article. CASP also helps to make the process simple by providing guidance notes for each answer. The checklists don't give a score but rather give an overall impression and allow you to discuss important points relating to the study. We therefore recommend using CASP checklists and discussing the study based on the points raised.

3.5.5 Notes on critical appraisal

You do not need in-depth critical appraisals of each individual article you find in your literature search; however, it is important to refer to the notes you have made on the articles, including any pertinent points raised while you have read the study. How you write depends on the purpose of your literature review, but we recommend taking notes under a pertinent heading in a set structure. This will make it easier to critically appraise a paper under the CASP headings. The following case study provides an example of how to appraise an article.

Case Study 3.2 Critical appraisal of a paper

In the following example, we utilise the CASP checklist for a systematic review. The paper we are examining is 'Mobile Phone Use and Glioma Risk: A Systematic Review and Meta-analysis'. This article has been published as an open access paper and so is free for anyone to view (https://pubmed.ncbi.nlm.nih.gov/28472042). The CASP checklist asked 10 key questions, and by answering these, you will be undertaking a global assessment of the quality of the paper.

#1 Did the review address a clearly focused question?
- The authors state the objective of their study is 'To investigate the potential association between mobile phone use and subsequent glioma risk using meta-analysis'. The authors chose to limit the study to the incidence of brain tumours rather than any other association with increased mobile phone usage and so have a focused question.

 # 2 Did the authors look for the right type of papers?
- The authors are evaluating an epidemiological question and wish to see if increased exposure to mobile phones leads to an increased incidence of glioma. Therefore the most appropriate studies are case–control studies, which the authors are indeed examining.

 # 3 Do you think all the important, relevant studies were included?
- Yes, the authors searched three major databases with appropriate terms to initially identify articles of interest. The authors then screened all results by reading the abstract of each study before final inclusion and also screened the references of these papers to identify any papers missed by their initial search strategy. The authors have also used logical and appropriate inclusion and exclusion criteria in this study.
- Another important strength of this study is that the articles included were not limited by the publication language. This strategy maximises the potential to find all of the important papers published on this topic.

#4 Did the review's authors do enough to assess the quality of the included studies?
- Yes. The authors performed an extensive quality assessment using a validated quality scale. This was performed by two independent members of

the authorship. Furthermore, an assessment of the potential sources of bias in each study, as well as a global measure of publication bias in all studies, was also undertaken.

#5 If the results of the review have been combined, was it reasonable to do so?
- The authors did combine the results of the systematic review into a meta-analysis. This was reasonable because there was no significant publication bias present in the published literature. However, for some of the main outcomes of interest, there was significant heterogeneity between studies. This limits the interpretation of these results, and so a meta-analysis in this case may not have been appropriate for all of the reported outcomes.

#6 What are the overall results of the review?
- Overall, there was a significant association found between mobile phone usage for more than 10 years and glioma risk (odds ratio = 1.44). The authors found increased odds of a low-grade glioma in patients with >10 years of mobile phone use, but there was no increased odds of a high-grade glioma.

#7 How precise are the results?
- The results of the study are quite precise, with relatively narrow confidence intervals from the results of the meta-analysis.

#8 Can the results be applied to the local population?
- This really depends on the local population we are discussing. The patients included in this systematic review were all from Europe, Southeast Asia, or the US. Therefore, it is unclear whether the results are valid in other areas. The authors have not provided an analysis of the sex of the participants or the ethnicity of the patients included in the studies. It is therefore not clear the exact population to whom this research applies.

#9 Were all important outcomes considered?
- Yes, in the context of this article the authors have broken down their analysis into important subgroups. This allowed, for example, not just brain tumours but those that were low-grade or high-grade. The authors also examined some specifics of mobile phone usage, such as which ear the phone was held to and how long the patients had been using a mobile phone.

#10 Are the benefits worth the harms and costs?
- This question isn't particularly relevant to this particular systematic review because the authors were examining an environmental exposure, namely mobile phone use. (In studies looking at a new drug treatment or a surgical intervention, this question would be more applicable!)

Chapter 4 **Ethics and the ethical application**

4.1 What is medical ethics and why is it important?

Ethics are the moral principles that guide one's behaviour in any given activity and in general conduct. As in day-to-day life, ethics help lay the moral groundwork for conducting our actions in a manner that is least harmful to the individuals involved and to society as a whole. In medical research, ethics are an indispensable facet of conducting research in a fashion that minimises damage and maximises welfare. The goal of research is to discover new knowledge and improve the lives of people globally. It is therefore essential that the process of conducting research in and of itself does not become a damaging process for those who take part in it, whether as researchers or as participants.

Generally, when you start to engage in any sort of medical research as part of a professional institute, you will have to agree to abide by the code of ethics that governs that institute, i.e. their ethical guidelines. While a code of ethics can vary depending on the institute, the specific field of research, and the sovereign nation you find yourself in, by and large all medical research ethical codes will have common principles among them. In this section of the book, we will discuss the main ethical considerations in medical research, the practical application of these ethics, and how to deal with conflicts that may arise as a result of ethical concerns.

4.2 Main ethical considerations in medical research

We will now review the major ethical considerations that arise in medical research and discuss each one briefly. These considerations are not nearly exhaustive, and as previously mentioned, some may vary from place to place. Be sure to review the specific ethical guidelines in your own place of research

How to Succeed in Medical Research: A Practical Guide, First Edition.
Robert Foley, Robert Maweni, Shahram Shirazi, and Hussein Jaafar.
© 2021 John Wiley & Sons Ltd. Published 2021 by John Wiley & Sons Ltd.
Companion website: www.wiley.com/go/foley/succeed

carefully. If you are found to be in breach of any of the ethical directions of your place of research, it could have serious implications for your research career.

4.2.1 Honesty

Probably the most important overarching ethical consideration to take into account is honesty. In all scientific communications, it is immensely important to honestly report data, results, methods and procedures, and publication status. Strive to never fabricate, falsify, or misrepresent data whether through intent or negligence. This includes colleagues, research sponsors, or the public.

4.2.2 Objectivity

Objectivity and honesty go hand in hand. Objectivity includes being honest with yourself and avoiding bias in experimental design, data analysis, data interpretation, peer review, personnel decisions, grant writing, expert testimony, and other aspects of research where objectivity is expected or required. Try to avoid or minimise bias or self-deception. Always disclose personal or financial interests that may affect your research.

4.2.3 Carefulness

Avoid careless errors and negligence; carefully and critically examine your own work and the work of your peers. It is vitally important to keep good records of research activities, such as data collection, research design, and day-to-day experimental procedures.

4.2.4 Openness

Share! Share data, results, ideas, tools, and resources with other researchers when appropriate. In addition, many online archives are now readily available for you to upload partial results, papers you did not have to time publish, or other data. Be sure to get permission and do your due diligence before using such an archive in this manner.

4.2.5 Respect for intellectual property

Honour patents, copyrights, and other forms of intellectual property. Do not use unpublished data, methods, diagrams, or results without permission. Give proper acknowledgement or credit for all contributions to research even when used for teaching purposes. Never ever plagiarise the work of others.

4.2.6 Confidentiality
Protect confidential communications, such as papers or grants submitted for publication, personnel records, and patient records or patient samples.

4.2.7 Responsible mentoring
Help to educate, mentor, and advise students. Remember always that a student is there first and foremost to learn. Do not treat students as simple workers or employees. Ensure they have a good learning environment in which they can gain the skills, knowledge, and techniques they need to become good researchers themselves. Promote their welfare. Enable and empower them to make their own decisions.

4.2.8 Respect for colleagues and personal conduct
Respect your colleagues and treat them fairly. Expect the same from them. Avoid discrimination against colleagues or students on the basis of sex, race, ethnicity, or any other factors not related to scientific competence and integrity. Report any violations of personal conduct you observe to the relevant personnel.

4.2.9 Social responsibility
Strive to promote social good and prevent or mitigate social harms through your research, public education, and advocacy.

4.2.10 Competence
Maintain and improve your own professional competence and expertise through lifelong education and learning; take steps to promote competence in science as a whole.

4.2.11 Legality
Know and obey relevant laws as well as institutional and governmental policies.

4.2.12 Animal care
Show proper respect and care for animals when using them in research. Do not conduct unnecessary or poorly designed animal experiments. Avoiding cutting corners where this might cause undue suffering to the animals under your care. Treat them with the respect and care sentient beings deserve.

Chapter 4

4.2.13 Human subjects protection

When conducting research on human subjects, minimise harms and risks and maximise benefits; respect human dignity, privacy, and autonomy; take special precautions with vulnerable populations; and strive to distribute the benefits and burdens of research fairly.

4.2.14 Informed consent

When conducting research involving human subjects who are capable of giving informed consent, each potential subject must be fully informed of the aims, methods, sources of funding, any possible conflicts of interest, the anticipated benefits and potential risks of the study, any discomfort it may entail, post-study provisions, and any other relevant aspects of the study. The potential subject must be informed of the right to refuse to participate in the study or to withdraw his or her consent to participate at any time without negative consequences.

Once the potential subject has understood the information, the physician or another appropriately qualified individual must then seek the potential subject's freely given informed consent, preferably in writing.

4.3 Practical ethical applications

So far we have discussed research ethics in a somewhat abstract manner through the discussion of some of the principles involved in research ethics. How does one apply the discussed principles in practical terms? How can a researcher identify when an ethical choice is to be made? Here we will give some examples of hypothetical cases in which ethical principles may apply.

Example 1

Dr M is conducting a study to observe the effects of a new drug on mouse models of neurodegeneration. The observation period is 2 weeks, and at the end of this period the mice are to be euthanized in order to carry out biochemical, histological, and cellular tests. Dr M was delayed in the onset of the experiment and is now a day behind schedule. As a result, the researchers will have to come in over the weekend to carry out the euthanization of the mice. Dr M feels that an extra day would not make much of a difference, so they decide to carry out the euthanization 1 day early and report the study as completed in the 2-week timeframe as originally planned.

Do you think this behaviour would be considered unethical?

Example 2

In the process of imaging a third nitrocellulose membrane for a western blotting experiment, Dr H accidentally loses the image files the researchers had taken of the membrane. Without quantifying them, the results looked by eye to be nearly identical to the previous two replicates they had carried out. As such Dr H decides to simply extrapolate and report the third membrane results with a reasonable estimate. Dr H then carries out a statistical analysis and finds the results to be significant.

Do you think this behaviour would be considered unethical?

Example 3

Dr R has been tasked with the taking and maintaining of records for a hospital study looking at post-operative care for a particular type of surgery. Dr R and the researchers have been diligent in their work throughout the study; however, one evening after completing their records for the day and heading home, Dr R realises they have left several files related to the study and patient records open on a desk in the staff lounge of the hospital. Dr R knows no one would take the files and decides to collect them in the morning.

What is wrong with this approach? What could Dr R have done differently?

Chapter 4

4.4 Dealing with conflicts in ethics

It may be that in your time in research you'll come across some ethical dilemmas or some ethics-related conflicts. Knowing how to deal with these issues is crucial to navigating your professional research career. Sometimes the issue may not be clear-cut and some time to reflect and think will be needed.

In general, there are a few common steps you can take to resolve an ethical conflict.

4.4.1 Identify and recognise the ethical conflict

In the first instance, being up to date and fully informed on your ethical responsibilities will allow you to identify when an ethical conflict has occurred and allow you to recognise its potential impact on your research. Sometimes it may be difficult to know when an ethical conflict has occurred or could occur in the course of your research. Many actions can be technically legal but still be against the ethical guidelines of your institute. Once you have clearly defined the ethical conflict you can move onto the next step.

4.4.2 Seek alternative courses of action

Sometimes the ethical conflict may be simply resolved by identifying and taking an alternative course of action if the original action was not crucial to the research. For example, if you identify that a conflict of interest is possible in your research due to financial commitments you or members of your research group have, it may be best to simply state clearly and openly what those financial commitments are once you publish your research. Otherwise it may be necessary to exclude any members with a conflict of interest from the study or end the financial commitment resulting in that conflict of interest. It is important for you to weigh up the feasibility of each option before coming to a decision.

4.4.3 Seek help or advice

If a feasible alternative course of action is not forthcoming, it may be best to consider seeking advice from senior researchers in your research group or department. Usually they will have faced similar issues in their research careers, or if not, they will know someone who has.

4.4.4 Decide on a definite course of action

After reviewing the situation, including referring to your institution's code of ethics, consulting with colleagues or superiors, and internal reflection, it should be time to make a decision. Remember – not taking any decision or not dealing with the ethical conflict in good time may also be unethical, even if it wasn't originally your fault. Always seek to deal with ethical issues well as soon as you become aware of them and well in advance of them becoming critical.

4.5 Ethical applications

Any research proposal involving animal or human subjects is subject to ethical approval, and the ethical considerations of that research must be clearly outlined and described for submission and approval to an ethics committee before the research can take place. It is important to take your time when filling in an ethical application, as they can be quite lengthy. If you are careless, you may have to wait for an extra period of weeks before your study receives ethical approval to begin data collection, which can be cumbersome and require you to radically change the timeframe of your study. Depending on the nature of your research and the specific guidelines of your institution, the exact content of an ethics application can vary. Some of the common features will include:

1. A full description of the aims, methods, and materials to be used in the study.
2. A detailed list of the number of subjects to be used (whether animal or human) and, where relevant, the timeframe for their participation, ages, sex, background, etc.
3. Explanation of how informed consent will be obtained and the details of what information will be included as part of that consent to the participants.
4. Details of pre-, during, and post-trial care for participants.
5. Details of any potential risks to participants and steps to be taken to minimise that risk.
6. Details of how participant data will be handled to ensure confidentiality. This includes written and digital data as well as biological samples from participants.

The online content section of this book contains a sample research proposal, patient information leaflet, and patient consent form as used in a successful ethical application.

Chapter 5 **Analysing your data**

Statistics has lots of practical elements and is not just theory. We will attempt to give you a grounding in medical statistics, but in order to truly learn statistics you will need to put in the time in the practical application of analysing your data. We also hope to arm you with the knowledge of which statistical analysis you need to perform for your own data, which is a big first step.

5.1 What I need to know and how to find it

Unfortunately, there is no magic bullet method to learning statistics, but there is a huge wealth of resources out there to help get you going. I believe it is worth having a grounding in how the calculations are performed; however, if this is not for you, then you can simply carry out the calculations needed to answer your particular research question. To begin, you will need to figure out how you are going to analyse your data.

There are a number of different statistical programs available to carry out your analysis, some of which are free, some expensive, and some very complex. Basic analysis can be carried out in an Excel spreadsheet, and there are also free software add-ins that allow for more detailed analysis to be done. A free software program for statistics is available, called R. If you have an abundance of time, I would highly recommend learning to code with R in the RStudio software. It is a very powerful tool, and you can download packages that enable you to do complex analysis. However, it is not very user friendly and will take time to learn. There are a number of other free statistical software programs available online to try, some of which are more basic but also easier to use. If you only need basic data analysis, a program such as SOFA Statistics may be perfect for you.

SPSS is often thought of as the workhorse statistical program in medical research. It is much more user friendly than R, and you can get started in it

How to Succeed in Medical Research: A Practical Guide, First Edition.
Robert Foley, Robert Maweni, Shahram Shirazi, and Hussein Jaafar.
© 2021 John Wiley & Sons Ltd. Published 2021 by John Wiley & Sons Ltd.
Companion website: www.wiley.com/go/foley/succeed

right away. There is a dropdown menu in the program for each statistical test you may wish to perform, and there are lots of easy-to-follow tutorials online, enabling you to carry out your analysis with minimum fuss. The problem, however, is cost. Hopefully, your library will have a copy of SPSS that you can use; otherwise, it is prohibitively expensive. Other programs such as SAS, MedCalc, GraphPad, and MathLab are similar to SPSS in that they have a cost associated with them. Sometimes you can avail of a free trial download so that you can try out the software.

See what software your department (hospital or university) has available. Visit the library and speak to the staff there. The library will often have access to a particular statistics program that has been paid for and you can use for free. The library may also offer group tutorials or one-on-one advice to get you started. This should be your first port of call before beginning your analysis.

Statistical analysis is a vital component of research, and there is often a statistician available to help you at your institution. Reach out and get in touch! Once you have tried the above methods to analyse your data, if you are having trouble or need specific help, talk to your statistics department. Your librarian may have more information on whether this kind of service is available.

If there is no source of help available to you, then I would recommend trying some of the easier analysis methods in Excel or with a free software program. The other option is to begin using R/RStudio, which will be tough at first but very beneficial in the long run.

Case Study 5.1 Learning statistics

When I took my first steps into research, it was as part of a 10-week student research programme. I had no previous experience in research prior to this, and the project I had applied for was a biostatistical one. I dedicated the first 4 weeks of my time on learning the basics of statistics. My first encounters with statistics came through statistics books at my university library and were closely followed by a series of videos from a free online learning resource called Khan Academy. The website teaches statistics from the very basics and is an excellent way to get an understanding of what statistics is and the theory behind it.

After I had an idea of what I was trying to achieve, I then began to try and analyse my data. I was analysing data from an Excel spreadsheet, and once I had worked out my categorical and continuous variables, I began to make tables to describe the data. I then started performing more detailed analysis using SPSS, which I had free access to through my university. My library had basic tutorials for starting to use the program, and I started with these. Although I was still very new to the use of statistics, I began to learn some basics of analysis using R, within the RStudio software. I found this difficult and time consuming, but I was, within a few days, able to carry out some analysis of my data. I also then learned to do some more advanced analysis in R, which was not available in SPSS, using online tutorials and guidance.

Following my 10-week research experience, I began a year of dedicated research time in the same group. And this is the point I really began to study statistics. I was fortunate to have a supervisor from the department of mathematics, who organised for me to receive regular tutorials from a PhD student in statistics. I began to learn about data management and organisation, and I began to learn new methods of data analysis, especially with the use of R. I found with R that the more I learned the more there was to learn. I undertook a diploma in statistics after this, which gave me a much greater understanding of the theory behind statistics and allowed me to gain a much deeper knowledge of the subject. I continue to use R for the majority of my statistical analysis now, and I continue to regularly learn new methods of data analysis.

5.2 Variables

Before we begin discussing how to analyse your data, it is important to know what type of data you are analysing. As mentioned in Chapter 2, variables can, in basic terms, be split into categorical and continuous data.

5.2.1 Categorical variables

Categorical data includes binary outcomes such as yes/no. For example, a patient can have a normal blood test or an abnormal blood test. Ordinal variables are another type of categorical data and are those where the data can take the form of certain values with a defined order. A commonly used ordinal variable in medical research is the Likert scale. This is a scale that ranges from 1 to 5 and can be used in a questionnaire, for example 'How much do you agree with the following statement. . .', where 1 is not at all and 5 is completely agree.

5.2.2 Continuous variables

Continuous variables are numbers that can take any value – for example, a patient's temperature. An important concept with continuous variables is that they can be converted into a categorical one if a cutoff is applied. For example, if a cutoff of 37° is applied to a group of patients' temperature data, and those >37° are abnormal, and those ≤37° are normal, we now have a new categorical binary variable. This is known as dichotomising a continuous variable.

5.2.3 Describing a continuous variable

To describe a variable in a cohort of patients we use certain measures that are dependent on the type of variable we are looking at. Mean and median are used to give us an idea of the middle value; they are known as measures of central tendency. The mean is the average value of a variable and is appropriate for continuous data that is normally distributed and does not have significant outliers. The standard deviation is also given to describe the spread of the data from the mean. The median is the middle value in your cohort, halfway between the largest and smallest value. The median is used for continuous data that is skewed or has outliers. The spread of the data is described using the interquartile range, which is the value of the 25th and 75th percentile of the data.

5.2.4 Displaying your variables

Table 5.1, taken from one of our publications [1], illustrates how to display these variables. Age, as a normally distributed continuous variable, is displayed with mean and standard deviation. Prostate-specific antigen (PSA) as a skewed continuous variable is described using the median and the interquartile range. Categorical variables can be easily described by the number and the percentage; the example in Table 5.1 shows the number of patients with a family history of prostate cancer. Ordinal variables can also be demonstrated in the same way, with each category listed in turn. The example Table 5.1 shows the grade of prostate cancer, an ordinal variable where Gleason 6 is the least aggressive grade of cancer and Gleason 10 the most aggressive.

Table 5.1 Patient characteristics.

Age, mean ± standard deviation	62.7 ± 7.6
PSA level, median (interquartile range)	5.2 (4.7–9.9)
Family history of prostate cancer, number (%)	206 (10.5)
Gleason score	
Gleason 6	454 (23%)
Gleason 7	426 (21%)
Gleason 8	179 (9%)
Gleason 9/10	94 (5%)

5.2.5 Normal distribution

Another important factor we need to consider is whether our continuous variables follow a normal distribution or not. Data that follows a normal distribution will have the appearance of a bell curve when plotted on a graph. Figure 5.1 illustrates the distribution of the ages in a dataset, which follows a normal distribution (Figure 5.1a), whereas the data for each patient's PSA level is skewed, or non-normal (Figure 5.1b). The method of deciding if data is normally distributed or not is firstly done with this visual inspection and secondly by formal testing. These tests for continuous variables such as age and PSA level are performed with either a Kolmogorov–Smirnov test and the Shapiro–Wilk W test. These can be carried out in your statistical software and are used in conjunction with your visual inspection. Tests for normality do not need to be carried out on categorical data.

5.2.6 Paired or unpaired data

Another important question you must ask yourself before analysing your data is whether or not it is paired or unpaired data. Paired data simply means that the variables you are comparing have been measured in the same patients. If you wanted, for example, to see changes in a patient's cholesterol levels over time, before and after an intervention (such as starting a new medication), then this is paired data, which requires different statistical tests to be applied. If, however, you have two different groups of patients, for example, a group with cancer and a group without, and are comparing their PSA levels, this is unpaired data.

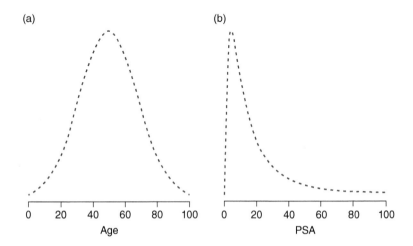

Figure 5.1 (a) Normal distribution. (b) Skewed distribution.

Chapter 5

To summarise our discussion on variables, firstly, Are they categorical or continuous? If continuous, are they normally distributed? And is the data paired or unpaired? Categorical data is summarised with numbers and percentages, while continuous data is summarised using the mean (if normally distributed) or median (if skewed). The variability or spread of the data is summarised with the standard deviation for normally distributed data and the interquartile range for skewed data.

5.3 Analysis of categorical and continuous variables in two groups

The statistical analysis carried out depends on the variables you are analysing. The test to use is summarised in Figure 5.2. If you have a continuous variable and are comparing two groups, this is done via an unpaired t-test (if normally distributed) or Mann–Whitney U test/Wilcoxon rank sum test (if non-normally distributed). If the data is paired, then a paired t-test and Wilcoxon signed-rank test, respectively, are used. Comparing a categorical variable between two groups is done via a chi-square test (or Fisher's exact test). However, if you are analysing paired data, McNemar's test is used.

5.3.1 The p-value
Once we have compared our variables with the above tests, a p-value will be produced. The p-value is a measure commonly used in the medical literature to assign 'statistical significance'. The p-value gives us an idea of how likely

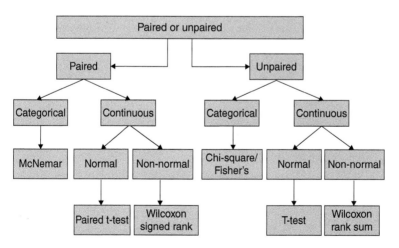

Figure 5.2 Flowchart describing the appropriate statistical test to use for each type of data.

the result is only down to random chance. A value of <0.05 (or <5%) is generally used in the literature as a cutoff for significance. An easy way to think about this is, for a p-value <0.05 the results would only occur at random less than 5% of the time, and so we assume that the result from our data is not due to chance. If the p-value is greater than 0.05, then we do not believe the result is 'real' because it could have occurred due to chance only. For example, suppose we measured the heights of 100 women who drive a blue car and 100 women who drive a white car and found that on average the drivers of blue cars are 3.5 cm taller than white car drivers. A t-test was carried out that demonstrated a p-value of 0.40, therefore this is >0.05, and our findings are not statistically significant. However, if our p-value was 0.01, this means that there is only a 1% chance of our result happening if there was truly no difference between the heights of the two groups. Therefore, we could confidently conclude that drivers of blue cars are indeed taller than white car drivers.

> **Case Study 5.2　Analysing and displaying your data**
> In Table 5.2, taken from one of our publications [1], we have two groups of patients, one with prostate cancer and one without. We have compared some continuous and categorical variables in R in these two groups of patients. We have listed the appropriate statistical test that was used and displayed our results.

5.4 Sensitivity and specificity

Sensitivity and specificity are essential components of research within the medical literature. They are often used to describe the performance of a particular diagnostic test, for example, a blood test. The key to understanding sensitivity and specificity is in a 2×2 contingency table. Let's take the following example: we wish to see how effective PSA is at discriminating between patients with and without prostate cancer. This analysis can be organised using a 2×2 table. This 2×2 table will allow for the calculation of the sensitivity and specificity of a test.

The study population is separated out into patients with cancer and those without cancer. We also separate out the population into those patients with a PSA level ≥ 4 and a PSA level < 4 (this is the traditional value at which prostate cancer was deemed more likely). It is important to note that we have now created a new categorical variable with our PSA levels, by dividing the patients into two groups. Our 2×2 table will look like Table 5.3.

The positives are those patients who were deemed positive by our PSA test, i.e. those with a PSA ≥ 4. And if those patients did indeed have prostate

Table 5.2   Patient characteristics.

	Prostate cancer	No prostate cancer	p-value
Age, mean ± SD	61.5 ± 6.9	63.8 ± 7.0	<0.01[a]
PSA level, median (interquartile range)	6.5 (5–8.9)	7.1 (5.4–10.7)	<0.01[b]
Family history, n (%)	78 (9%)	128 (11%)	0.19[c]

[a] Student t-test.
[b] Mann–Whitney U test.
[c] Chi-square test.

Table 5.3   2 × 2 table: test outcomes.

	Group 1 (patients with cancer)	Group 2 (patients without cancer)
Patients with a PSA level >4	True positives	False positives
Patients with a PSA level <4	False negatives	True negatives

Table 5.4   2 × 2 table: numeric test outcomes.

	Group 1 (patients with cancer)	Group 2 (patients without cancer)
Patients with a PSA level >4	80	50
Patients with a PSA level <4	20	50

cancer, then this is a true positive result. However, if a patient with a positive PSA test did not have cancer, this would constitute a false positive result. Conversely, those patients with a PSA level <4 and who had prostate cancer represent the false negatives, while those who did not have cancer are the true negatives. The better a test performs in a particular population is determined by maximising the true results and minimising the false results.

For example, suppose we have 100 patients with prostate cancer and 100 patients without prostate cancer in our study population. Each patient has a PSA blood test, and we calculate how many patients have a PSA ≥4 or <4. Creating a 2 × 2 table for this example allows us to calculate our sensitivity and specificity (see Table 5.4).

5.4.1 Sensitivity

The sensitivity of a test is a measure of how well the test performs in the patients who have a disease (in this case prostate cancer). In other words, how well does the test diagnose prostate cancer when it is actually present?

A highly sensitive test diagnoses most cases of a disease, thereby maximising its true positive results. A highly sensitive test also does not miss many cases of a disease and minimises false negative results. The sensitivity of a test is reported as a percentage, as shown in the following example:

$$\text{Sensitivity} = \text{True Positives}/(\text{True Positives} + \text{False Negatives}) \times 100$$

$$\text{In our example, sensitivity} = 80/(80 + 20) \times 100 = 80\%$$

5.4.2 Specificity

The specificity of a test is a measure of how well the test performs in patients who do not have disease. We are interested in the column of patients in Group 2 in Table 5.4. Another way of thinking of specificity is how well this test rules out disease in patients who do not have a disease. A very specific test will rarely label a patient who does not have a disease as a positive result, minimising the number of false positives. A highly specific test will not diagnose patients with a disease when they do not have it, maximising the number of true negatives. Specificity is calculated as follows:

$$\text{Specificity} = \text{True Negatives}/(\text{True Negatives} + \text{False Positives}) \times 100$$

$$\text{In our example, sensitivity} = 50/(50 + 50) \times 100 = 50\%$$

5.4.3 Interpretation

Our data demonstrates that in our population of 200 patients, 100 with cancer and 100 without, PSA has a sensitivity of 80% (or 0.80) and a specificity of 50% (or 0.50). What this means is that in patients with prostate cancer, a PSA test will be positive in 80% and negative in 20%. In patients without prostate cancer, a PSA is positive in 50% of patients and negative in the other 50%. We can therefore think of the PSA test as having a good sensitivity but only moderate specificity. The better a test performs, the higher both the sensitivity and specificity will be.

5.5 Positive predictive value and negative predictive value

It might strike you that sensitivity and specificity may not be incredibly useful if you have already performed a test on a patient in clinical practice. Suppose you are a doctor and you have performed a PSA test to try to aid in the diagnosis of prostate cancer. However, you do not know if the patient has prostate cancer or not, and so you cannot directly apply sensitivity and specificity to your patient. Suppose the patient's PSA result is 5. This is greater than 4 and so is a 'positive result' on a PSA test. There is another metric we can calculate from our 2×2 table to help us in this situation, called the positive predictive value.

The positive predictive value (PPV) of a test is a measure of how likely a patient with a positive test is to have a certain disease. In this scenario, the PPV is a measure of how likely it is that a patient with an abnormal PSA test result will have prostate cancer. It is calculated as follows:

$$\text{Positive Predictive Value} = \text{True Positives} / \\ (\text{True Positives} + \text{False Positives}) \times 100$$

The PPV in this scenario would be $80/(80 + 50) \times 100 = 62\%$.

If we apply this result to our patient in practice, this means that because he has a positive PSA result, he has a 62% chance of having prostate cancer.

On the other hand, if our patient has a PSA value of 2, then this is a negative result. The negative predictive value (NPV) of PSA, from our table, is as follows:

$$\text{Negative Predictive Value} = \text{True Negatives} / \\ (\text{True Negatives} + \text{False Negatives}) \times 100$$

The PPV in this scenario would be $50/(20 + 50) \times 100 = 71\%$.

For our patient with a negative PSA test, we can extrapolate his likelihood of being disease free is 71%, and so his risk of having prostate cancer is 29%. In this way, the PPV and NPV can help us in clinical practice more readily than the sensitivity and specificity values if the test has already been performed.

5.6 Receiver operating characteristic curves

A receiver operating characteristic (ROC) curve is another important concept when it comes to the statistical analysis of a test. This is essentially a plot of sensitivity versus specificity. From this we can calculate the area under the curve (AUC). The AUC value gives us an idea of how well a variable or test performs in predicting a particular outcome. In an ROC curve (Figure 5.3), the 45° line represents an AUC of 0.50 (which can be thought of as 50%). This is the performance expected by flipping a coin, i.e. a coin would have a 50/50 chance of guessing correctly heads. The broken line in Figure 5.3 achieves an AUC value of 1.0. This is a perfect outcome and is the aspiration of any test; however, in reality this is very difficult to achieve. The ROC curves for two other variables are illustrated, with AUC values of 0.85 and 0.70, demonstrating two imperfect tests; however, both are better than a coin flip.

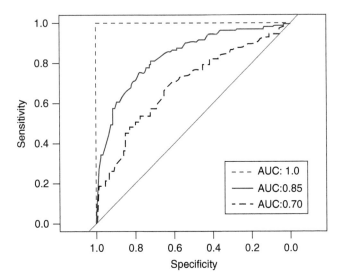

Figure 5.3   Receiver operating characteristic curves.

The way an ROC curve works is by plotting the sensitivity and specificity or a particular variable along all of the available cutoffs. To explain this, think again about the previous example in which PSA was used as a categorical variable with a cutoff value of 4 to decide a positive and negative test. However, if we want to analyse the relationship of PSA as a continuous variable and whether a patient has cancer or not (without dichotomising PSA into a categorical variable), we can use an ROC curve. In Figure 5.3, PSA was the variable used to produce the ROC curve with an AUC of 0.70. Using the ROC allows for a single metric to describe the performance of PSA, at every possible cutoff level, in the prediction of prostate cancer rather than reporting sensitivity, specificity, PPV, and NPV separately.

5.6.1 95% confidence intervals
When reporting AUC values for a variable, it is best to include the 95% confidence intervals. The 95% confidence interval is a statistical concept that is commonly reported and important to understand. Essentially, it gives the range of values you would expect a result to fall into 95% of the time if you repeated the measurement on different groups of patients repeatedly. Different variables with different AUC values can also be compared to each other, and a p-value can be derived to demonstrate whether the difference in AUC values is statistically significant or not.

Case Study 5.3 Comparing two variables with ROC curves

In one of our publications [2], we compared the performance of two blood tests in the diagnosis of prostate cancer, one of which was PSA and the other prostate health index (PHI). We did this by reporting the AUC values and the 95% confidence intervals. We also compared the two ROC curves in R and reported the p-value for the difference.

The PHI score was the most predictive of prostate cancer in terms of discriminative ability, with an AUC for the PHI score of 0.78 (95% CI 0.71–0.84) in the prediction of PCa compared with an AUC of 0.70 (95% CI 0.63–0.77) for PSA. This difference was statistically significant (p<0.01).

5.7 Logistic regression analysis

A relatively more complex method of analysis we will touch on is logistic regression. Logistic regression is used to predict a binary outcome, such as whether a patient has cancer or not. Logistic regression can be used to create a model that takes into account only one variable, such as PSA. It can also include a number of different variables, so instead of only using PSA to predict whether a patient has prostate cancer, we can also use age and whether the patient has a family history. As you can see, family history is a categorical variable. This can also be included in a logistic regression model. This model can then be used to give each patient a probability of having prostate cancer from 0 to 100%. Logistic regression models are becoming commonplace in the medical literature, as researchers attempt to predict patients who have a disease based on their clinical characteristics.

When we create a logistic regression model, an odds ratio is calculated for each variable that was used to create the model. An odds ratio gives us an idea of the likelihood of an outcome. It shows the odds of a particular outcome in one group compared to another. For example, in a study we could look at the rates of lung cancer amongst smokers and non-smokers, and we may find an odds ratio of 10. This means that the odds of a patient who smokes having lung cancer are 10 times higher than the odds of a non-smoker. Our logistic regression model will also calculate a p-value for each variable, which signifies if the variable is a significant predictor of the outcome. We can also compare logistic regression models using the same method we used earlier, namely ROC curves and AUC values.

Case Study 5.4 Logistic regression

In the following example, we have created a logistic regression model to predict the likelihood of a patient having a large brain tumour based on his or her symptoms and the examination findings of the doctor [3]. This is a method of identifying which variables are predictive of a large tumour size. The results demonstrated that a patient suffering with headache or with facial weakness was significantly more likely to have a large brain tumour, with odds ratios of 3.1 and 5.3, respectively. The results were displayed as in Table 5.5, with 95% confidence intervals and p-value.

Table 5.5   Logistic regression results.

	Odds Ratio (95% CI)	p-value
Headache	3.1 (1.8–5.4)	<0.01
Facial Weakness	5.3 (2.7–10.6)	<0.01

5.8 Other types of analysis

There are many other methods of data analysis that you may come across and indeed need to use in order to answer your research question.

5.8.1 Comparing two continuous variables

Two continuous variables, such as patient age and PSA level, can be compared using correlation analysis. This analysis will examine the relationship between the two variables in the total cohort, i.e. it cannot compare groups. If one variable increases with the other also increasing, this is a positive correlation. The correlation coefficient (denoted by 'r'), shows the strength of the relationship, with a value of 0.8–1 demonstrating very strong correlation. Correlation can also be negative; for example, if PSA were to decrease as patient age increased, this would be a negative correlation. This may be a moderately strong negative correlation, with an r = −0.5. Table 5.6 shows one method of interpreting an r value.

Two continuous variables can also be analysed via linear regression. Linear regression functions in much the same way as logistic regression; however, the outcome data in linear regression is continuous as opposed to a binary (yes/no) outcome. Linear regression can also be performed with multiple variables. A linear regression model will return an R-squared (R^2) value, which explains how much of the variability in your outcome can be predicted by the model. R^2 values will range from 0 to 1 (0–100%), and the higher the value, the more the variation in outcome is explained by the model.

Table 5.6   Interpretation of the correlation coefficient (r).

Correlation coefficient (r)	Interpretation
(±) 0–0.2	Very weak correlation
(±) 0.2–0.4	Weak correlation
(±) 0.4–0.6	Moderate correlation
(±) 0.6–0.8	Strong correlation
(±) 0.8–1	Very strong correlation

5.8.2 Comparing three or more groups

You may have three groups of patients and want to compare a variable across these groups. For example, we had three groups of patients who had undergone either surgery, radiotherapy, or neither and we wished to compare quality of life outcomes in these groups [4]. This is performed with an analysis of variance (ANOVA) test. The ANOVA test is analogous to the t-test for groups of three or more. It compares the means in each group and produces a p-value.

5.8.3 Inter-observer variability

If you wish to examine the agreement between two observers, you can use Cohen's kappa or the intra-class correlation coefficient (ICC). Cohen's kappa is used for categorical variables, for example, if there are two observers who label a number of wrist x-rays as 'fracture' or 'no fracture'. However, if you are using continuous variables, such as two observers who are recording patients' blood pressure readings, the ICC can be used.

5.8.4 Time to event data

You may have time to event data. In other words, you may have recorded the number of days until a patient dies. This type of data is commonly used in studying the efficacy of an intervention, such as how much time passed between each patient's surgery and each patient's death. This is often termed 'survival analysis' and can be depicted with a Kaplan–Meier curve. We can also create a regression model using the variable we have collected for each patient to attempt to predict our outcome, i.e. whether the patient survives or not. This is called a Cox proportional hazards model and is the equivalent of a logistic regression model in this setting. It will produce a hazard ratio for each variable rather than an odds ratio.

5.9 How to present your results

Table 5.7 demonstrates which type of graph or table to use when displaying your data. These are the most commonly used methods, although there are others, as we will discuss in the next case study. Always be on the lookout for new and interesting ways to display your data!

Table 5.7 Displaying data.

Data	How to display your data
Two continuous variables	Scatterplot
Two categorical variables	2 × 2 table
One categorical and one continuous	Boxplot, ROC curve
Several groups and one continuous variable	Bar chart, pie chart, boxplot

Case Study 5.5 Radar chart

It is always worth thinking about how best to display your data for poster presentations, oral presentations, or publication. When we were analysing our data for quality of life in patients with acoustic neuroma, we knew we could display our results in a table or a bar chart, but we were open to new methods of presenting our data that would help the results to stand out. We had quality of life outcomes in three groups of patients and in seven different domains. Displaying all of this data in a bar chart would not have been visually appealing, and so we decided to use a radar chart. This allowed us to illustrate the quality of life in our three groups of patients (those treated with surgery, radiotherapy, or a conservative strategy) and the quality of life in each domain. It also allowed for a comparison between the groups to be seen visually with relative ease. Figure 5.4 illustrates the quality of life in each domain from 0 to 100.

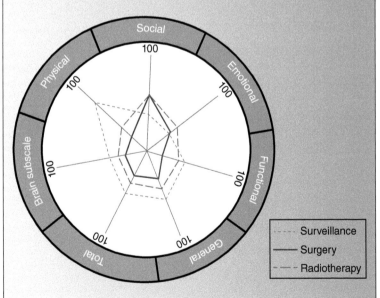

Figure 5.4 Radar chart.

5.10 Conclusion

Statistical analysis is not something to rush through. However, if you take some time to invest in understanding how to analyse your data you will be rewarded for your efforts. This chapter aims to give you a starting point to work from so that you can perform the correct analysis, or if you cannot, you will be able to find the best method to help you on your way.

References

1. Foley, R.W., Maweni, R.M., Gorman, L. et al. (2016). European randomised study of screening for prostate cancer (ERSPC) risk calculators significantly outperform the prostate cancer prevention trial (PCPT) 2.0 in the prediction of prostate cancer: a multi-institutional study. *BJU Int.* **118**: 706–713. https://www.ncbi.nlm.nih.gov/pubmed/26833820.
2. Foley, R.W., Gorman, L., Sharifi, N. et al. (2015). Improving multivariable prostate cancer risk assessment using the prostate health index. *BJU Int.* **117**: 409–417. https://www.ncbi.nlm.nih.gov/pubmed/25847734.
3. Foley, R.W., Shirazi, S., Maweni, R.M. et al. (2017). Signs and symptoms of acoustic neuroma at initial presentation: an exploratory analysis. *Cureus* **9**: e1846. https://www.ncbi.nlm.nih.gov/pubmed/29348989.
4. Foley, R.W., Maweni, R.M., Jaafar, H. et al. (2017). The impact of primary treatment strategy on the quality of life in patients with vestibular schwannoma. *World Neurosurg.* **102**: 111–116. https://www.ncbi.nlm.nih.gov/pubmed/28284966.

Chapter 6 Conferences and presentations: the next step in the research journey

Conferences are a wonderful opportunity to present your work. They are an integral step in the research journey and allow you to showcase your work to other researchers. To attend a conference, you will need to have your study planned, your data collected, and your analysis performed. This is the chance to bring together your findings into a coherent structure and to start thinking about how to present those findings.

Conferences are also an excellent opportunity to see what other research is being performed, a chance to talk to other researchers and be inspired with new ideas for future areas of research. It is also a great time to speak to other researchers about issues you have had, to get advice and perspective on how others may have dealt with similar problems, and to find researchers for collaborative projects in the future. Presenting your work offers a great chance to fine-tune your ideas for writing a paper for publication and can often offer up interesting points for the discussion section of your paper.

6.1 Types of conferences

In general, the types of meetings will be split up into local, national, and international. Local meetings can vary from your research laboratory monthly meeting to your hospital's annual research day or to regional meetings in certain specialties. National conferences are generally much larger affairs and may include a larger array of topics. These meetings are an ideal way of disseminating your research and finding others in your country who have similar research interests. International conferences can be quite daunting in terms of their size, with thousands of attendees and hundreds of sessions taking place. These types of meetings are melting pots for different researchers from around the world and can be a fantastic learning experience. Often when presenting at an international conference,

How to Succeed in Medical Research: A Practical Guide, First Edition.
Robert Foley, Robert Maweni, Shahram Shirazi, and Hussein Jaafar.
© 2021 John Wiley & Sons Ltd. Published 2021 by John Wiley & Sons Ltd.
Companion website: www.wiley.com/go/foley/succeed

world experts can be chairing or judging your session, and so it is a great opportunity to talk to the best people possible. The conferences you will attend will vary depending on your location and your field of research. However, the basic principles are the same, and you should aim to work your way up from local through to national and on to international meetings. Speak to your supervisor about which conferences are the most appropriate for your research.

6.2 Prices and prizes

Other factors to consider include the cost of attending, the prizes on offer, and the publication of abstracts. Many conferences will offer free or reduced prices to attend for students or young researchers. Speak to your supervisor about funding, as often research teams will have funding to attend conferences if you are presenting. Another important consideration are the prizes on offer. Some conferences offer excellent cash prizes that will allow you to fund your trips, whereas others offer a free trip to another conference as a prize. The main prizes will be a poster presentation prize and an oral presentation prize. It can be difficult to prepare your poster or talk in order to win a prize; however, they are an excellent incentive to prepare to the best of your ability so that you have the greatest chance of winning. When deciding on conferences to submit your work to, look for those that offer prizes in categories that will apply to you, for example, student prizes. The other consideration is whether or not abstracts will be published. It is preferable to have a published abstract because it is another method of getting your research out there and visible. Check what journal your abstract will be published in and be sure to keep a copy for your records.

Chapter 6

Case Study 6.1 Conferences

I began my research career in the field of prostate cancer. The first conference I attended and submitted my research to was a local meeting for my university. From there I attended national meetings in Ireland, the Irish Urology Society annual conference and the Irish Association of Cancer Research, on the advice of my supervisor. Because Ireland is a relatively small country, I also attended national conferences in the UK, such as the British Association of Urological Surgery annual conference. I then submitted my work to the large international conferences in the field of urology, the European Association of Urology annual conference and the American Urological Association annual conference.

6.3 Abstract submission

Once you have decided on which conference to submit to, you will need to write an abstract. An abstract is a short (usually 200–250 words) summary of your research. It will be judged by a panel and a decision made on whether the abstract is suitable to be accepted for the conference.

Look through the accepted abstracts from previous conferences, which will usually be published on the conference website. This will give you a good idea of the standard of submission and the scope of research that is accepted, and it will also provide you with a good idea of how your abstract should be structured. The abstract submission guidelines will have specific rules for how to lay out your abstract, but for a scientific abstract in general, it will take the form of a title, introduction, methods, results, and conclusion. It should generally be quite trouble-free for you to write an abstract for submission, as most of the groundwork will already have been done. The title of your study, introduction, and methods will be included in your research proposal and analysis plan carried out at the beginning of your study. The results will have been analysed after collection, and so the conclusion should be the only part that requires some new attention.

6.4 Title

The title should sum up your research, but try not to be too long-winded. Another good tip is to try not to include a question in the title. Be brief and to the point.

6.5 Introduction

The introduction is an outline of the background information to your study. Try to describe why the disease process you are studying is important. Next, outline the main objective of your study.

6.6 Methods

The methods section is where you outline the patient cohort or the model organism included in your study. It also details what information you collected, or in a laboratory setting which techniques were used. You also outline what analysis you performed and what statistical methods were utilised.

6.7 Results

The results section highlights the main findings from your data analysis. Try to only pick one or two key points for the abstract because the word count is quite limited. In some cases, a table or figure can also be submitted, and this is an excellent opportunity to demonstrate your results without eating into the allocated word count. Check the submission guidelines to see if this is possible.

6.8 Conclusion

The conclusion is essentially a reiteration of the main objective of the study. Describe the outcome of the study and what your results show. If possible, try to finish with a statement of what the next step is from here. That may take the form of a statement or a recommendation for future research based on your results.

Examples of abstract submissions for conferences are given in the following case studies.

Case Study 6.2 Abstract 1
Title
Analysis of Pro[-2]PSA; A Novel Biomarker That Significantly Improves the Detection of Prostate Cancer in a Referral Population.

Introduction
In order to effectively select patients for prostate biopsy, more accurate biomarkers of disease are needed. The objective of this study was to analyse the clinical utility of a novel biomarker, pro[-2]PSA, in order to inform the decision for prostate biopsy in an Irish cohort of men.

Methods
The serum of 250 men from three tertiary referral centres with pre-biopsy blood draws was analysed for tPSA, fPSA, and pro[-2]PSA. From this the phi score was calculated (pro[-2]PSA/fPSA)*√tPSA). Calibration plots and receiver operating characteristic (ROC) analysis as well as decision curve analysis were utilised to ascertain the potential utility of the phi score.

Results
The phi score was well calibrated in this cohort, demonstrating good correlation between predicted probabilities and actual outcome. The area under the curve (AUC) for the phi score was 0.72 for the prediction of prostate cancer and 0.78 for the prediction of high-grade prostate cancer (Gleason $\geq$ 7), compared to 0.62 and 0.70 for tPSA. Decision curve analysis demonstrated net benefit of the phi score over its entire range of risk probabilities.

Conclusion
The measurement of pro[-2]PSA can increase the accuracy of risk calculation in each individual patient, thereby helping to better inform the decision for prostate biopsy in a referral population.

Chapter 6

Case Study 6.3 Abstract 2
Title
The Impact of Primary Treatment Strategy on Vestibular Schwannoma Patient Quality of Life

Introduction
To assess the quality of life (QoL) in a representative sample of vestibular schwannoma patients and to ascertain the differences in outcomes associated with distinct management strategies.

Methods
Vestibular schwannoma patients attending a tertiary referral centre were asked to complete the FACT-Br Questionnaire, which assesses QoL in five domains: physical, social, emotional, and functional and a brain-cancer-specific domain. Results were analysed in the overall cohort and in surgery, stereotactic radiosurgery, and conservative management subgroups. The relationship between patient clinical characteristics and QoL outcome was also analysed by univariable and multivariable logistic regression.

Results
There were 83 survey respondents with an average age of participants of 57 years and a mean follow-up of 4.9 years. QoL was statistically significantly lower in the surgery subgroup within the physical QoL domain (p = 0.039). However, there was no significant difference in overall QoL between the three subgroups of surgery, radiosurgery, and conservative management (p = 0.17). A poor QoL outcome was associated with the number of symptoms at diagnosis, greater tumour size, and a surgical management strategy.

Conclusion
The QoL within this patient cohort was extremely variable in each management group, mirroring the heterogeneous natural history of this disease process. QoL in vestibular schwannoma patients cannot be predicted based on management strategy alone, but a poor QoL outcome is more likely in patients with larger, symptomatic tumours that are surgically treated.

Case Study 6.4 Abstract 3
This abstract was submitted to a Thoracic Society conference and takes a slightly different form. This abstract is of a case report, and the submission guidelines differed from that of a scientific study. Case reports and case series are often accepted into conferences, and there can be a separate prize section for interesting patient cases.

Title

Metastasectomy of a Solitary Lung Melanoma of Unknown Primary in a Patient with Type 1 Neurofibromatosis

Introduction

Malignant melanoma is a common skin neoplasm bearing poor prognosis when presenting with metastases. Rarely melanoma metastases present without an identifiable primary cutaneous lesion despite exhaustive workup.

Case report

We describe the case of a solitary lung metastasis in a 65-year-old man with neurofibromatosis type 1 without an identifiable primary tumour. A computed tomography (CT) guided biopsy of the mass was obtained, and histological examination demonstrated a deposit of large nucleated epithelioid cells with pigment, positive for S100 and Melan A. Physical examination and positron emission tomography – computed tomography (PET/CT) imaging to establish the primary lesion were complicated by the presence of numerous PET-avid superficial neurofibromas, and therefore, no primary lesion was identified. Our patient was managed by video-assisted thoracoscopic metastasectomy. Three months after his original presentation, a primary melanoma was identified in the patient's jawline, hidden by his beard. He succumbed to his illness 11 months after initial presentation.

Conclusion

Melanoma of unknown primary should be investigated with appropriate imaging studies; however, the importance of a thorough physical examination cannot be overemphasised. Bearing in mind the close association and causative relationship of NF1 and malignant melanoma, a thorough physical examination of a patient who presents with a metastatic deposit of melanoma must be carried out in an effort to identify the primary lesion and to expedite appropriate management.

Chapter 6

6.9 Poster presentation

6.9.1 Poster design

Making a poster can be quite an enjoyable experience and a chance to get a bit creative. However, it can be daunting to make one if you haven't done so before. We have provided a number of templates in the online content with this book. Have a look at these examples, and use the layout to create your own poster. The poster will follow the layout of your abstract, with the title, introduction, methodology, results, and conclusion sections. Be sure to make the title nice and large so it can easily be read from a distance. At the top of the poster, next to the title include the logo of your hospital, university, or institution. At the bottom of the poster, you can include logos of any collaborating institutions. I believe in including lots of images in a poster, as in essence it is a visual display, and a picture tells a thousand words. Also, it will be difficult to hold the attention of the viewer for very long, so a good image will get the message of your poster across much quicker.

6.9.2 Poster presentation sessions

Some poster presentation sessions will come with a designated presentation slot, of 2–5 minutes in duration. These quick presentations are sometimes tricky, with not enough time to properly discuss your research. However, they can be excellent practice and are another chance to really get to know your data inside out. The presentation may take the form of two or three judges who will allow you to tell them about your research, or they may interrupt and ask lots of questions. Questions can be difficult to answer on the spot, but just try your best. Afterwards, quickly make a note of all of the questions you were asked during your presentation. If you didn't have a good answer at the time, think of what the best answer would be. Chances are you will be asked a similar question again in the future – in particular, when your paper is under peer review. Remember that posters and podium presentations are a stepping stone to submitting a work for publication. These questions can be excellent sources of ideas for what to include in the discussion section of your paper, making for a stronger submission. We will discuss writing a paper in more detail in the next chapter.

6.10 Podium presentation

When submitting, you will generally have a choice of submitting for a poster or a podium presentation. The podium presentation is certainly more effort; however, it is always best to try to submit for an oral presentation. Because it requires more effort and time to prepare your presentation, it will stand to you. You will have a better understanding of your research and you will need to make slides, which will mean you will be better prepared when it comes to writing up your research for publication. You are also more likely to be asked questions and receive detailed feedback from judges and researchers in the audience. You can then use this to improve your study, as we previously discussed.

Practically speaking, when it comes to an oral presentation a rule of thumb is to use one slide per minute of your presentation. This will depend on the content of your slides, of course, but one pitfall to avoid is trying to cram too much into your presentation and running over time. Judges can be particularly strict with timing rules, so it is better to be short and leave time for questions rather than going over time. Again, as for poster presentations, try to use images to illustrate your main points where possible. Having too much text on your slides will mean that people spend their time reading instead of listening to you talk.

Include your main results in the form of graphs if you can, and use a laser pointer to draw attention to the important findings. However, be careful if you are using this approach that you don't turn your head too far away from the microphone so that you can no longer be heard. A set of example oral presentations has been included in the online content with this book. Take a look at these examples and notice the number of slides, layout, and use of images. Use these templates as pointers to make your own presentation.

Chapter 6

Chapter 7 **Writing a paper**

To illustrate how to write a paper, we will be referring to one of our own publications throughout this chapter [1]. This paper examines a blood test and risk models for the prediction of prostate cancer. It is available for free online, and the link is included in the reference section of this chapter. We highly recommend downloading the paper and reading through the sections in full as you read this chapter to reinforce the concepts. We will now discuss each section of a paper in turn, starting with the title.

7.1 Title

The title of your paper should already be written from your study protocol. However, we will again mention that in your title it is important to be relatively brief and to include the main point of your paper. The ideal title

---

Case Study 7.1 Title

Interestingly, the original title for our paper was much more long-winded than the final one. A reviewer of the paper asked us to change to a shorter title, and it was definitely much better after the change.

Our original title was:

Analysis of the Performance of a Prostate Cancer Clinical Prediction Model Incorporating Pro[-2]PSA (p2PSA) in the Form of the Prostate Health Index (PHI)

This was updated and changed for the published paper:

Improving Multivariable Prostate Cancer Risk Assessment Using the Prostate Health Index

---

How to Succeed in Medical Research: A Practical Guide, First Edition.
Robert Foley, Robert Maweni, Shahram Shirazi, and Hussein Jaafar.
© 2021 John Wiley & Sons Ltd. Published 2021 by John Wiley & Sons Ltd.
Companion website: www.wiley.com/go/foley/succeed

should portray the most amount of information about your paper with as few words as possible. You will need to include the disease process or patient population in your title and what you will be examining in your study. The study design, i.e. cohort study or randomised trial, can also be included.

7.2 Abstract

The abstract is a short summary of your study. It will usually consist of defined subsections just like the full paper. Writing an abstract is covered in Chapter 6, and when it comes to writing your paper, the abstract will generally have already been written during submission for presentation at conferences. It is important that your abstract has the crucial information you wish to get across to your reader because commonly this is the chance to entice the viewer into reading the full paper.

Case Study 7.2 Abstract

Examples of abstracts were given in Chapter 6. The abstract should outline the objective of the study, the study cohort and number of patients, the main result or outcome of the study, and a general interpretation of the results. Here is the abstract from our paper.

Objectives

To analyse the clinical utility of a prediction model incorporating both clinical information and a novel biomarker, p2PSA, in order to inform the decision for prostate biopsy in an Irish cohort of men referred for prostate cancer assessment.

Patients and methods

Serum isolated from 250 men from three tertiary referral centres with pre-biopsy blood draws was analysed for total prostate-specific antigen (PSA), free PSA (fPSA), and p2PSA. From this, the Prostate Health Index (PHI) score was calculated (PHI = (p2PSA/fPSA)*$\sqrt{tPSA}$). The men's clinical information was used to derive their risk according to the Prostate Cancer Prevention Trial (PCPT) risk model. Two clinical prediction models were created via multivariable regression consisting of age, family history, abnormality on digital rectal examination, previous negative biopsy, and either PSA or PHI score, respectively. Calibration plots, receiver operating characteristic (ROC) curves, and decision curves were generated to assess the performance of the three models.

Chapter 7

Results

The PSA model and PHI model were both well calibrated in this cohort, with the PHI model showing the best correlation between predicted probabilities and actual outcome. The areas under the ROC curve for the PHI model, PSA model, and PCPT model were 0.77, 0.71, and 0.69, respectively, for the prediction of prostate cancer (PCa) and 0.79, 0.72, and 0.72, respectively, for the prediction of high-grade PCa. Decision-curve analysis showed a superior net benefit of the PHI model over both the PSA model and the PCPT risk model in the diagnosis of PCa and high-grade PCa over the entire range of risk probabilities.

Conclusion

A logical and standardised approach to the use of clinical risk factors can allow more accurate risk stratification of men under investigation for PCa. The measurement of p2PSA and the integration of this biomarker into a clinical prediction model can further increase the accuracy of risk stratification, helping to better inform the decision for prostate biopsy in a referral population.

Chapter 7

7.3 Introduction

The literature review that you have written will set the stage for your introduction. If people who knew absolutely nothing about the topic were reading your paper, they should, by the end of the introduction, be able to understand what topic you are looking at, why you are looking at it, and what question you plan to answer. You should also explain the relevant literature on the topic that led to the question being asked.

Start off by explaining the disease process you are studying with some background information. In our paper, we start by giving some basic epidemiology about prostate cancer:

> *Prostate Cancer (PCa) is the most common solid organ malignancy amongst men in Ireland and is second only to lung cancer as the single largest cause of cancer-specific mortality. Ireland has one of the highest incidences of PCa in Europe and, according to published incidence rates from 2012, was over 50% higher than the EU average.*

Next you need to describe the background to your study, which essentially means summarising the findings from the literature that frame the need for your research question. This is the reason, or the rationale, behind your study. In our paper, we discuss how prostate cancer is diagnosed with a biopsy and how the clinician decides on the need for a biopsy:

The gold standard for the diagnosis of prostate cancer is a prostate biopsy. The decision on who to send for this procedure is a difficult one. The clinical judgment and recommendation to proceed with a prostate biopsy hinges upon assessment of risk factors such as PSA, digital rectal examination (DRE), a positive family history of prostate cancer, age, previous prostate biopsy as well as the patient's life expectancy, psychological status, and the patient's wishes.

We also set the scene by discussing how risk calculators offer a way to bring together patient's risk factors in the best way possible:

Through the systematic use of patient risk factors, in the form of prostate cancer clinical prediction models, risk stratification can be standardised and used to guide clinical decision making. . .

And next we briefly mention that a new blood test (biomarker) has been shown to have the potential to improve prostate cancer diagnosis, although we don't go into too much depth at this point in the introduction. We discuss these results in more detail in the discussion section of the paper:

A novel biomarker, p2PSA, has been shown to be preferentially expressed in malignant prostate tissue and to correspond to aggressiveness. Several papers have demonstrated the potential benefit of p2PSA measurement in men under investigation for prostate cancer.

The final portion of the introduction should discuss the specific objective(s) of your study or the hypothesis you are trying to test. We believe that this should be explicitly stated in the introduction, such as in our paper:

We hypothesise that the measurement of p2PSA and its incorporation into a logistic regression model along with other clinical parameters will improve risk stratification in an Irish cohort of men referred for prostate cancer assessment.

7.4 Methods

The methodology section of your paper needs to be a detailed description of how the study was conducted. The level of detail should be such that it would allow someone to reproduce your study. There are a number of important points that need to be mentioned in this section, including the patient population included in the study, the outcomes you are measuring in the study, how these outcomes were acquired, and how your results were analysed. It can be broken down into subsections, as we have done in our paper, to describe the patient cohort, the laboratory methods, and the statistical methodology.

To start your methods section of the paper, describe the patient population and the time period over which the study was conducted:

> *The study cohort consisted of 304 patients who were identified from an ongoing multicenter risk stratification study of men referred to an Irish Rapid Access Clinic for the assessment of prostate cancer between April 2012 and August 2014.*

Describe how you chose your patient population, how you identified the study cohort, and decided who was included in the study and who was not (i.e. eligibility and exclusion criteria):

> *These men were selected based on the availability of a pre-biopsy biobanked serum specimen. . .Men younger than age 40 or those with a previous diagnosis of PCa were excluded. The final cohort consisted of 250 men after the exclusion of patients with inadequate serum volume or without full clinical information.*

Next, outline clearly what outcomes you are measuring and how you collected this outcome data. For our paper, we needed to give a detailed description of how we collected and analysed a patient's serum to measure our variables:

> *Nine millilitres of blood was collected directly into a vacutainer blood collection tube containing serum clot activator and centrifuged at 1,500g for 10 minutes at room temperature. . .Patient serum was analysed for total PSA (tPSA), free PSA (fPSA), and p2PSA on the Beckman Coulter DxI800 Unicel Immunoassay system.*

Describe the statistical methods used to analyse your data. Also include the statistical software you used to look at this. In our paper, we detailed our basic statistical analysis and also the creation of logistic regression models (risk calculators) from our data:

> *Basic statistical analyses of the study population's characteristics were performed using the unpaired Student's T-test and the Wilcoxon rank sum test for continuous variables, while Pearson's Chi-squared test was performed for categorical variables. . .*

Two models were created by multivariable logistic regression. One of which incorporated tPSA along with age at biopsy, abnormality on DRE, family history of PCa, and a previous negative biopsy. . .

All statistical analysis was carried out using the R software programme and the relevant statistical packages.

7.5 Results

To start the results section, give the demographic information for your study cohort. This can take the form of a table and is the most basic description of your study population. It allows the reader to see what sort of population has been studied and whether this is applicable to the clinical context in which he or she is working. This includes details like the number of patients, sex, average age, and other clinical characteristics based on your specific study cohort. For example, in the case of our prostate cancer study we described the number of patients with prostate cancer and those without, whether there was a positive family history, whether the patients had had a previous biopsy before, etc. We listed this as a table in our paper. We also took the opportunity to display our basic statistical tests in the same table, separating the study cohort into the two groups of prostate cancer and no prostate cancer.

In our paper, we did not describe much of the patient's demographic information at the beginning of the results section but rather directed the reader's attention to the relevant table to look at:

Of the 250 patients, 112 (45%) were diagnosed with PCa on biopsy and 77 (31%) were diagnosed with high-grade disease. Table 2 shows the clinical characteristics of the patient cohort.

Now you can write down the main results of your paper, the one that answers the objective of the study. This should also be displayed in a graph or diagram as appropriate.

In our paper, we analysed the use of a new blood test panel in prostate cancer diagnosis (PHI score). We outlined how this PHI score performed compared to the usual blood test used in clinical practice (tPSA):

Analysis of the available biomarkers demonstrates that the PHI score is the most predictive of biopsy outcome in terms of discriminative ability, with an area under the curve (AUC) for the PHI score of 0.71 in the prediction of PCa compared to an AUC of 0.62 for the tPSA value that was available to the clinician (p<0.01).

Our main objective was to analyse the performance of the PHI score in a multivariable model for the prediction of prostate cancer, and so we discuss

Chapter 7

these results next. We compared the performance of this PHI model to a model using tPSA, which is a blood test that is readily available in clinical practice:

> *The AUC for the PHI model in the prediction of PCa was 0.77 and was significantly greater than that of the PSA model, AUC=0.71 (p<0.01).*

If you have performed any secondary analysis or subgroup analysis, include this next. In our prostate cancer patients, we decided to perform a subgroup analysis on the patients that had previously undergone a prostate biopsy:

> *AUC value [using the PHI model] for the prediction of prostate cancer was 0.85 in our repeat biopsy patients (n=60). This represents an improvement from AUC values of 0.70 for the PSA model (p<0.01)*

Another important consideration in writing the results section of your paper is how you will display the main results. It is important to make good use of tables and figures throughout your paper. Depending on the results you have, it may be appropriate to use bar charts, scatterplots, ROC curves, etc. Decide on the best graph to display your data and include this in the paper. For example, in our prostate cancer paper, we had two multivariable models, the PHI model and the PSA model. In order to illustrate how these two models differed in the prediction of prostate cancer in our cohort, we decided that a scatterplot would be the most effective method:

> *Figure 3 illustrates the probabilities of the model without the novel biomarker calculation (PSA model) and the new probabilities given by the model incorporating the PHI score (PHI model). There is appreciable scatter from the 45-degree line, indicating that the PHI model is potentially useful in patient counselling, as its risk probabilities can be seen to vary markedly from those of the PSA model.*

7.6 Discussion

This section is composed of a summary of the main findings of your paper, and you should attempt to place these findings within the broader knowledge already available from the literature. A lot of this can be taken from your previous literature review, although be sure to check again for any new publications that are relevant to your study prior to submitting your paper for peer review.

There are two main approaches that can be taken when writing the discussion section of your paper. You can summarise the literature on a paper-by-paper basis, or you can use each paragraph in your discussion to make a specific point and include the literature relevant to that point in each paragraph.

In our prostate cancer paper, we took the 'point-by-point' approach. We had a few choice points we wished to make in our discussion, and we made our references based on these. One of the main points we wished to make was that the use of a novel blood test to predict prostate cancer should be included in a multivariable model to analyse how well it could perform. Here is how we discussed this topic and included our references:

> *Several papers examine PHI in isolation and do not form predictive models [26, 27], or indeed form these models and neglect one or more important methods of statistical analysis [23]. . .[It is wrong to] analyse a biomarker's clinical utility without the creation of a multivariable model and drawing a comparison to a model that does not include this novel biomarker [16].*

We also summarised the main findings of the paper:

> *The PHI score is a more discriminant biomarker than PSA, has superior calibration, and has a superior net benefit; therefore, by using PHI-based risk stratification, urologists will be in a position to make a more informed decision in each patient.*

Address the limitations of your study at the end of the discussion, explaining any potential sources of bias or weaknesses of the study that were unavoidable. One such potential source of bias in our paper was that some of the blood tests had been performed at different hospitals and using different machines. Another limitation of the study was a possible selection bias. Here is how we addressed these issues:

> *One potential confounding factor, which may help to explain, in part, the variation in performance of the PSA model and PHI model, is that the measurement of PSA available to the clinician pre-biopsy was taken across the three institutional sites participating in the study.*
>
> *We acknowledge several limitations in this study. The sample size is relatively small and the study population was ethnically homogenous. Because recruitment was based on patient willingness to participate, it is impossible to exclude a selection bias.*

7.7 Conclusion

The conclusion is essentially a short review of the main results and main point of your paper. Conclusions may include the potential clinical impact of your findings or may make a recommendation for future areas of research. In the conclusion of our paper, we again make reference to the importance of an accurate diagnosis in patients under investigation for prostate cancer, and we summarise our main results:

> *In order to risk stratify patients pre-biopsy and direct resources towards those patients most in need, thus reducing the risk of a biopsy to those who do not require the procedure, all possible tools in the urologist's armamentarium must be examined. This includes novel biomarkers for PCa and a multivariable approach to risk stratification. The PHI score improves significantly upon PSA and when incorporated into a multivariable model, patient risk stratification is further improved.*

7.8 References

As mentioned in the literature review chapter (Chapter 3), there are software applications that are an ideal way to keep track of your references. Using these tools, you can simply insert your references as you write the paper, and a reference list is automatically compiled at the end of your paper. We highly recommend you find the ideal software tool for you, as this will make formatting your references quite simple. The style of your references will depend on the journal you are submitting to.

When referencing, it is vital that you have referenced correctly and avoided plagiarism. Once you are happy with your paper, check through your paper and each reference to double-check you are citing the correct paper. It is not uncommon for authors to submit a paper for peer review and to have used an incorrect reference. Try to avoid this pitfall because it is can lead to a poor outcome from the reviewers.

7.9 Sending to seniors for review

Once you have completed your paper, it is important to send the manuscript to the other authors so they can make changes or comments. Speak to your supervisor first, as he or she will be the senior author and may wish to be sent the first draft of the paper before the other authors. It is essential that you are extremely well organised when sending your paper for review. Save your paper as version 1, and save each author's returned manuscript by using his or her initials and the version number. If you do this it will be easy to keep track of the latest manuscript, but if you are not organised, it can quickly turn into a nightmare, especially if there are a lot of reviewers and a lot of edits. Most authors will track their changes in the Word document, but if this is the first time you have worked with someone, then do remind the person to track changes, and it will be much easier for you to incorporate all of the author's updates into updated versions of the paper. Once all of the changes have been made, your paper will be ready for submission!

Reference

1. Foley, R.W., Gorman, L., Sharifi, N. et al. (2016). Improving multivariable prostate cancer risk assessment using the prostate health index. *BJU Int.* **117**: 409–417. https://www.ncbi.nlm.nih.gov/pubmed/25847734.

Chapter 8 **How to get published**

8.1 Which journal?

There are a huge number of medical journals that you can submit your work to and that will potentially publish your article. It can often be difficult to decide on what journal is the best choice for your paper. The first port of call should be to discuss this with your supervisor; however, as with everything in research, if you do a bit of work before seeking help, you will be in a better position to make a decision. There are a number of factors to consider when deciding on where to submit.

8.1.1 The scope and readership of the journal

This is arguably the most important point when selecting your journal. You will want to publish your work in a journal that is most likely to reach the target audience for your paper. So, if you write a paper that looks at the imaging features of a musculoskeletal disease process, you will want to target radiologists, orthopaedic surgeons, or rheumatologists. You can do this by targeting a journal that caters to these clinicians. Before deciding on where to submit, look through the articles that have previously been published by each journal to see if your research fits in with the scope of the journal.

8.1.2 Indexing

Another important factor to consider, which ties in with the readership of the journal, is indexing. Be sure to check what databases are listing the articles published in each journal you look at. MEDLINE (Medical Literature Analysis and Retrieval System Online) is one of the most commonly used databases, the search engine for which is PubMed. If a journal is not listed on MEDLINE and other common databases, your research will be far less accessible and much less likely to be found by other researchers and clinicians.

How to Succeed in Medical Research: A Practical Guide, First Edition.
Robert Foley, Robert Maweni, Shahram Shirazi, and Hussein Jaafar.
© 2021 John Wiley & Sons Ltd. Published 2021 by John Wiley & Sons Ltd.
Companion website: www.wiley.com/go/foley/succeed

8.1.3 Impact factor

The impact factor of a journal is a metric that looks at the average number of references that are made of the papers published in a journal. It is not a perfect measurement tool, but it is a surrogate marker for how important a particular journal is and how much influence the journal has within the field of medical research. It is preferable to publish your paper in a journal with a higher impact factor, as this means the article is more likely to be read. Impact factors are often quoted on each journal's website, and a full list of official impact factors for all journals is published annually by Thomson Reuters™. Before meeting with your supervisor, try to find a few journals that may be suitable for your research and note down their impact factors.

8.1.4 Open access publication

Open access articles are free to be read by anyone, and there is no need to pay for access. If your article is not behind a paywall, this will make your article as accessible as possible, and it can be read by as wide an audience as possible. In order for a journal to be able to publish open access, the cost is often transferred to the authors of the article. This is not always necessary, as some journals have no charges for open access publication.

Open access publication can be an excellent way to provide access to the latest research to those who cannot afford it, and the cost is often covered by research grants. However, you must be vigilant of some journals with large fees for publication. They are often easy to recognise, and these journals may contact you by email and have no recognised readership or impact factor.

Depending on your place of work, your institution may have a publishing agreement with certain journals. This can be incredibly helpful in opening up your article to possible open access publication. Many journals with open access charges will offer a waiver if you are from certain countries, so if applicable this is worth investigating in each of the journals of your shortlist.

Chapter 8

Case Study 8.1 Selecting a journal for submission

In Chapter 7, we outline how our prostate cancer research paper was written. However, once the paper was written (and in many cases, well before the writing begins), we needed to select the most suitable journal for our article. This is not a decision that I made on my own, rather I consulted with my supervisor and other senior authors before making our decision. One of the most important aspects in the selection process was the readership of the journals. The article in question included a laboratory aspect to it, in that we were measuring biomarkers from the blood samples of each of our patients. Many of the authors were from a basic science background, hence some of the journals we were considering submitting to, such as *The Prostate* or *Prostate Cancer and Prostatic Diseases*. However, we decided that because of the translational aspect of the paper, taking the laboratory research to a clinical setting, we wished to submit to a journal with more of a clinical focus.

The most prestigious of these journals was *European Urology*, with the highest impact factor of any urology-related journal and one of the highest impact factors of any surgical journal. However, we felt that this journal was likely out of reach, as similar studies had already been published in this journal with larger patient numbers than our own article. The other journals that we considered included the *Journal of Urology*, *Urology*, *World Journal of Urology*, and the *British Journal of Urology International*. All of these journals had similar impact factors, but the standout choice was the *British Journal of Urology International*, because it is commonly read by urologists and researchers in urology in both Ireland and in the UK, which is where the study was conducted. We felt that publishing in this journal helped us reach the best audience for our paper.

Another factor that played into our decision was that my supervisor had worked with the editorial board for the journal advising on translational research studies (such as the one we had conducted), and so he knew the journal would be interested in our article. Our department also had a subscription to this journal, and so we each received the latest issue every month and were therefore aware of the articles published in this journal. Interestingly, while the study was being conducted, I met the journal editor at a conference in London. I introduced myself and we spoke about the journal readership and the scope of the journal. I was convinced after this discussion that the journal would be suitable for our goals with the article. Another important factor was the opportunity to publish in open access, which would allow our paper to be read by anyone for free.

8.2 Authorship

Another important topic before the submission of your paper is the authorship. It is important that each author has contributed to the article in some way, although invariably the first author will do the majority of the work. The senior supervisor is the final author, and he or she will often oversee the whole research process and do the majority of the editing of the manuscript. Ask your supervisor which authors to include and how to order them. After the first author, the order of authorship will often be decided by how much work each person has contributed to the research. The second author is often another more junior member of the research team who did the next most work in the project, and the order will continue in this way. Be sure to ask the authors when you are sending around the paper for editing how they would like their name included in the article. Many journals look for the academic qualifications of each author, so it may be worthwhile asking for this information as well.

8.3 Getting your paper ready for the journal

Once you have your paper written, reviewed by the other authors, and a decision made of the journal, you are ready to submit! Each journal will have specific author guidelines on its website. Use these author guidelines to help format your article in the correct way before you submit. The guidelines will provide you with a step-by-step process to follow to ensure you submit your article correctly. There may be a word count you need to adhere to; there may be a limit on the number of references you can provide or a limit to the number of authors.

The guidelines will also detail the abstract word count and the abstract headings. The headings for the paper will generally be the same between journals but may have minor variations. Some papers, for example, will want a 'Conclusion' section separately, while others will want a final 'Discussion' section only. You will also need to submit a list of keywords with your article; these allow the article to be found more easily when searched for on a database. These keywords are published with each article, so consult similar papers or the papers you are referencing in your article for ideas on the best keywords.

The guidelines will also outline the style of referencing the journal uses, and you will need to adhere to this. This can be made far easier through the use of automated referencing software, as discussed in Chapter 3.

A cover letter is often required or allowed with a submission. This is merely a letter to the editor of the journal outlining in brief the paper you have submitted. It is a courtesy that we feel is well worth including in your submission. A sample cover letter has been included in the online section that accompanies this book.

Another important piece needed for submission is a title page. What is needed on this page may vary slightly but will follow a general format between journals. Usually it will include the title of your article (hence the name!), the authors, author affiliations, details for the corresponding author, keywords for your article, and a conflict of interest statement. Again, a sample title page is available in the online content section.

When you are finished formatting the paper for your chosen journal, it is important to proofread your article carefully. It can be extremely useful to ask for help with this. Ask someone you trust; this does not have to be a co-author because the proofreader is checking for mistakes in the spelling and grammar of your manuscript rather than the scientific merit. Be meticulous in this step.

Submission takes place online, and there will be an opportunity to check your work before finally submitting. Make sure you have everything you need for submission in a folder, organised and named appropriately before you start uploading, as it is likely you will need to make small changes throughout the process.

8.4 Dealing with reviewer comments

Once you have submitted your article, you can relax! The process is generally not too fast, and there may be quite a few weeks and sometimes months before the paper has been peer reviewed. Generally, one of the members of the journal editorial board will send your paper to two or three reviewers, who will read your paper, write down their comments, and submit their response to the editor. The reviewers will usually have one of four courses of action they can recommend to the editor: firstly to accept your article with no changes, secondly to accept the article with minor changes needed, thirdly to accept the article with major changes needed, or fourthly to reject the article.

In many cases, you will need to make revisions to your paper before it will be accepted, and unfortunately the paper may be rejected.

If accepted with changes required, you will have to respond to the reviewers and make changes to your article. This may be small changes to the text or changes to the figures or tables you have provided, or it may require more work in the form of new data collection, more data analysis, or major reworking of the text. In the following case study, we will show you an example of the reviewer comments we received for a paper and how we responded.

Case Study 8.2 Response to reviewers

We submitted a case series of children with abdominal non-Hodgkin's lymphoma to a paediatric surgical journal, and it was accepted following revisions [1]. Here are the reviewer's comments and the reply I wrote back following discussion with the senior authors. As you will see, sometimes you will need to fight your corner and defend your article, while on other occasions you will thank the reviewer for a suggestion and incorporate it into your article.

Reviewer 1: Comments to the author

This manuscript presents three cases with nonspecific abdominal symptoms of lymphoma. The authors address the importance of awareness of lymphoma as a differential diagnosis when we confront the prolonged nonspecific abdominal symptoms. This report is interesting and well written. However, the occurrence of lymphoma including NHL on abdomen is relatively common. There are several reviews of lymphoma series presented abdominal symptoms and acute abdomen. In my view, *Paediatrics International* is not a proper journal for this case report. This manuscript should be submitted elsewhere.

Response to reviewer 1
We thank the reviewer for their comments. The authors believe that *Paediatrics International* is indeed the most appropriate medium for the dissemination of the findings of this case series for reasons outlined below. The scope of *Paediatrics International* 'aims to encourage those involved in the research, practice and delivery of child health to share their experiences, ideas and achievements. . .for the benefit of children everywhere.' The author has highlighted the need to evaluate abdominal NHL in the differential diagnosis of children presenting with an abdominal complaint, especially those with unexplained or prolonged symptoms. It is acknowledged that although the incidence of abdominal NHL is common, the potential to overlook this diagnosis on initial presentation certainly exists. We have provided three interesting examples of such presentations and indeed these patients were delayed an accurate diagnosis as NHL was initially overlooked.

Although case series of abdominal NHL do exist as the reviewer has mentioned, these illustrate common presentations and fail to highlight the potential mistakes associated with the diagnosis. Moreover, none illustrate as effectively the spectrum of disease presentation, which can mislead the physician. Other published work also fails to illustrate the presentations that may masquerade as another possible disease entity. The unique value of our paper is that it offers an educational standpoint from which we hope lessons will be learned for physicians managing children with abdominal NHL to avoid delay in diagnosis. The vital point of this paper can be summarised with the concept: if it's not in your differential diagnosis, then you won't diagnose it. We believe this is in keeping with the focus of this journal.

Reviewer 2: Comments to the author
This is an important case report for alarming the delay of the accurate diagnosis for NHL patients with unusual clinical presentation. I recommend this manuscript for publication in *Pediatrics International* after getting author's answers to my following questions.

#1: How many paediatric NHL patients were treated in your institution during the treatment of these three patients? I would like to know the rate of the patients with unusual clinical presentations among the paediatric NHL patients.

#2: How many days did it require from the date of biopsy to start chemotherapy? Were there any surgical complications in the biopsy or resection of these patients? The authors emphasised the importance of providing quicker initiation of chemotherapy and also the advantage of laparoscopic biopsy. Therefore, the actual data should be presented in the case report.

#3: Related with #2, was the resection necessary in case 1 as an initial treatment? As far as reading this case presentation, the surgical resection was possibly avoided in case 1. Let me know the author's opinion.

Response to reviewer 2
We thank the reviewer for his/her comments and have attempted to address each one in order below.

#1: The patients in this paper were diagnosed between 2011 and 2014. The latest cancer figures for Ireland for paediatric NHL showed 27 children were diagnosed in 2010. All of these patients were treated at our institution, as it is the national paediatric oncology centre. We can extrapolate from the latest figures that these three unusual presentations make up approximately 3% of patients diagnosed with NHL.

#2: Date of biopsy to chemotherapy was between 1 and 3 days for these three patients. No biopsy-related surgical complications occurred. The paper has been updated to include this information as per the reviewer's suggestion.

#3: That is a very interesting question. And it is a question that is up for debate, in that many paediatric surgeons/oncologists will give you very different answers. In paediatric NHL, surgical resection can be undertaken. Some will recommend this be performed if it can be done with adequate surgical margins [2], while others only recommend excision if another indication for surgery exists [3]. In the absence of a randomised control trial (which is unlikely to be performed in this population), it will be down to the expert opinion of the surgeons and oncologists taking care of each individual patient. In the opinion of the authors, surgery should not be performed owing to the high sensitivity of paediatric NHL to chemotherapeutic protocols alone, and the potential surgical morbidity to the child can therefore be avoided.

Reviewer 3: Comments to the author
The authors described three cases of abdominal NHL in children with various clinical manifestations challenging early diagnosis.

#1: As they mentioned in the study, it has been well known that abdominal NHL can lead to a broad spectrum of clinical signs and symptoms. Therefore, the reviewer doubts that the three reported patients, especially case 1, had really 'unusual' presentation of abdominal NHL. The authors should explain what is the 'unusual' point of those cases.

#2: Although the authors suggested the importance and limitation of imaging studies in general, they did not clarify those issues associated with the three NHL patients, especially case 2 and 3. What caused the delay of diagnosis in case 2 and 3?

#3: Presenting images of the three cases in figures separated by modalities (US, CT, MRI) without timeline makes this report hard to understand. Figures should not be separated by modalities but by cases according to the text. Moreover, each figure needs arrows, marks, or text to help us find the lesion and orientation.

#4: Was there ileal or appendiceal perforation in case 2? If so, what was the strategy of treatment for patients with both NHL and intestinal perforation?

#5: Although the authors implore open-minded care of paediatric patients with abdominal symptoms in order to reach the diagnosis of NHL, it is not something new worth publishing. They should go through their diagnostic process with a critical eye and illustrate their recommended strategy of early diagnosis for children with NHL based on review of their experience.

Response to reviewer 3

#1: The unusual point of these cases is that the diagnosis was not easily discernible, was mistaken for another diagnosis, and the physical examination and/or initial imaging erroneously endorsed the incorrect diagnosis. As regards case 1, the patient had a history of intussusception and a palpable mass in the right upper quadrant. Initial ultrasound imaging supported the diagnosis of intussusception. It was only at the time of laparoscopy that the initial diagnosis was discarded and biopsy confirmed NHL.

#2: The initial imaging studies in all cases were misleading, and when we suggest the importance of imaging, we refer to the correct interpretation of these images in children with NHL. Although difficult, there are a few diagnostic features that can easily be missed. These features are mentioned in the discussion. The delays in diagnosis in case 2 and 3 were both down to misdiagnosis. Case 2 was diagnosed with an appendiceal perforation, treated with IV antibiotics; however, when the patient failed to respond, a repeat CT scan was requested. At this time, a node with calcification raised suspicion for NHL, and a raised LDH all but confirmed the diagnosis. The patient was then biopsied. As for case 3, the delay in diagnosis of this child was again down to a misdiagnosis on initial imaging. CT scan demonstrated what was believed to be an inflammatory mass in the abdomen. Again, due to prolonged symptoms beyond the scope of the original diagnosis, further imaging was obtained – this time in the form of an MRI. The patient's diagnosis was reconsidered following this imaging.

#3: We have changed the images for this paper so that the figure corresponds to each case as requested by the reviewer so as to enhance the reader's understanding of the case series. In response to the reviewer's suggestion, we have included arrows in the figures in order to direct the reader towards the area of pathology more readily.

#4: The patient in case 2 had an appendiceal perforation. However, following diagnosis of NHL, there is a question of whether or not the mass should be resected. Because it would be difficult to fully resect the area of involved bowel with clear margins and because the operative field would be complicated because of the intestinal perforation, the decision was made to proceed to chemotherapy and to continue IV antibiotics (2 weeks, then switched to oral) to treat the peritoneal infection.

#5: This is a very important comment, and we thank the reviewer for pointing this out. We have added a recommendation for early diagnosis of paediatric abdominal NHL to the discussion in line with the reviewer's suggestion. After careful consideration, we believe the salient points to be:

i. Lower threshold for LDH serum testing in cases of an abdominal mass, even if imaging suggests the mass to be inflammatory;
ii. To consider the limitations of basic imaging in its capacity to discern what appears to be simple diagnoses;
iii. Radiologists must be thorough in the examination of imaging for potential signs of NHL (as outlined in the discussion);
iv. Always keep NHL in one's differential diagnosis;
v. Be aware of the various presentations that abdominal NHL can take, including some of those that are unusual (as outlined in the case presentations).

8.5 Dealing with rejection

Rejection is a common problem that you will encounter at some point if you are submitting papers for publication. It can be quite a disappointment, but try not to let it get you down. The next step is to take any author comments that you think will improve your paper and include them prior to your next submission. Discuss with your supervisor the next journal to submit to and start the process again!

Case Study 8.3 Acoustic neuroma paper submission [4]

As discussed in Chapter 2, I had decided to carry out a study into the quality of life of patients with acoustic neuroma, a type of brain tumour. The study spanned over a 2-year period from the idea, through the research proposal, ethical approval, data collection, and data analysis. Following presentation of the data at conferences, it was time to write up the paper for publication. We had originally decided to submit the paper to an ear, nose, and throat (ENT)-focused journal, as it had a high impact factor and had published papers on quality of life in acoustic neuroma in the past. The paper was submitted and underwent peer review. There were three reviewers who each made comments to the paper, which were used to improve the paper before an amended version was submitted. This process happened again a second time, with further reviewer comments and revisions, but ultimately the paper was unfortunately rejected. However, using the improvements we had made to the article, we submitted again, this time to a neurosurgery-focused journal, and were accepted for publication following some minor revisions [4].

References

1. Foley, R.W., Aworanti, O.M., Gorman, L. et al. (2016). Unusual childhood presentations of abdominal non-Hodgkin's lymphoma. *Pediatr. Int.* **58**: 304–307. https://www.ncbi.nlm.nih.gov/pubmed/26670157.
2. Laver, J.H., Kraveka, J.M., Hutchison, R.E. et al. (2005). Advanced-stage large-cell lymphoma in children and adolescents: results of a randomized trial incorporating intermediate-dose methotrexate and high-dose cytarabine in the maintenance phase of the APO regimen: a Pediatric Oncology Group phase III trial. *J. Clin. Oncol.* **23**: 541–547.
3. Pulte, D., Gondos, A., and Brenner, H. (2008). Trends in 5- and 10-year survival after diagnosis with childhood hematologic malignancies in the United States, 1990–2004. *J. Natl. Cancer Inst.* **100**: 1301–1309.
4. Foley, R.W., Maweni, R.M., Jaafar, H. et al. (2017). The impact of primary treatment strategy on the quality of life in patients with vestibular schwannoma. *World Neurosurg.* **102**: 111–116. https://www.ncbi.nlm.nih.gov/pubmed/28284966.

Chapter 8

Chapter 9 **Writing a case report**

Though close to the bottom of the hierarchy of evidence, case reports and case series are a crucial part of the body of medical knowledge. They can often provide the only evidence base, particularly in subjects where it is difficult to conduct experimental trials, such as some disciplines of surgery and most commonly, pertaining to rare diseases. For a medical student or junior doctor, they are an excellent opportunity with which to practice one's skills in writing a paper and to submit for publication. Indeed, the authors of this book managed to publish a number of case reports as medical students, through which we were able to demonstrate our interest in research to our seniors as well as have some credentials with which to impress them.

There are further benefits, as at many levels in your career, published case reports will count as publications and, therefore, you will be awarded points for them for job applications. This can be a difference maker in applying to some competitive specialties, such as surgical training positions. The extra points can also be helpful in obtaining a job in a competitive geographical area, even in less competitive specialties.

9.1 How to begin

Before writing a case report or case series, there are a number of questions you need to consider.

9.1.1 Why this particular case?

This is the most important factor to consider. Why do you want to write about a particular story? The fact that your consultant or registrar has suggested it is not sufficient. The answer you give here will also be useful when you are writing up your case report's discussion section, as you often need to justify why you believe this case report should be published. There are a variety of reasons

How to Succeed in Medical Research: A Practical Guide, First Edition.
Robert Foley, Robert Maweni, Shahram Shirazi, and Hussein Jaafar.
© 2021 John Wiley & Sons Ltd. Published 2021 by John Wiley & Sons Ltd.
Companion website: www.wiley.com/go/foley/succeed

you or your team might wish to write about a particular subject, and we find the best way to think about them is as per the *British Medical Journal* (BMJ) Case Reports submission portal, which lists the following as case types: New Disease, New Diagnostic Procedure, Novel Treatment, Rare Disease, Reminder of Important Clinical Lesson, Unexpected Outcome, Unusual Association of Diseases/Symptoms, and Unusual Presentation of More Common Disease. There are other case types such as Global Health and Medicine in the Humanitarian Sector, should you be interested in these.

Using this list, you can consider in which category your case fits and tailor it accordingly. For example, if you are writing about a rare disease, it will be important, during your literature review, to find out how many cases of that rare disease are reported in the literature.

9.1.2 Is it the most efficient use of my time?

Whilst a case report is quicker and easier to write than the process of planning and running a study, it is somewhat less prestigious and often will not contribute as much to the body of medical knowledge. If, at the same time, you have the opportunity to participate in a randomised controlled trial, for instance, perhaps this would be a better use of your time. You must also consider your experience – if you have already published a number of case reports, unless this case report contributes significantly to the body of knowledge or it is relating to a topic that is close to your heart, perhaps it would be more prudent to focus on gaining experience with an evidence type you are yet to try, e.g. systematic review or meta-analysis.

9.1.3 Does it need to be written?

Before committing to writing a case report (or indeed, committing to any research project), it is advisable to carry out a quick preliminary literature review. It does not need to be as extensive as described in the literature review section of this book; however, it does need to furnish you with information on how much evidence is already out there regarding your subject of interest. In case reports, where you are not necessarily making a significant addition to the body of medical knowledge but rather reporting an interesting case, this is even more important, as it can show you whether or not your case will be redundant and superfluous.

Case Study 9.1 Should I write this case report?

As a surgical trainee in otolaryngology, I treated a patient who had developed an abscess in his frontal bone during a bout of sinusitis. This is often termed a Pott's puffy tumour, after Dr Percival Pott, an English surgeon who initially

Chapter 9

described it in the eighteenth century. In the classical description of this pathology, there is osteomyelitis of the frontal bone and often a defect in the anterior plate of the frontal bone. The peculiar thing about this case was that there were no signs of osteomyelitis on radiological imaging, and there was no defect in the anterior plate.

As I considered writing about this novel presentation, I performed a quick literature review on subperiosteal abscesses of the frontal bone and found that it was not a common occurrence. However, there was already a significant amount of literature describing this finding, including an explanation of how the infection spreads through drainage of the diploic veins from the frontal sinus to the subperiosteal layer. I thus abandoned the plan to write about this case, as there was no need for it and it would not be adding to the body of medical knowledge.

9.2 Preparing to write the case report

9.2.1 Case notes

It is advisable to begin with a draft of the case in chronological order – noting down, in a logical order, the presenting complaint, the history, examination findings, investigation results, diagnosis, and treatment. To write this fully and in requisite detail, you will likely need a copy of the patient's notes, so it is prudent to request these notes from Medical Records ahead of time so that you have them available. However, many healthcare providers now have electronic patient records that make this process quick and painless. Ensure you include all investigation results that may be pertinent – especially laboratory and radiological studies.

This initial draft should have as much detail as possible – you aren't going to publish this draft, but it ensures that you know all the facts of the case and will be able to answer any questions from your seniors and other departments from whom you might seek help, and do so in a clear, confident, and convincing way. It is also prudent to keep, as journal peer reviewers can ask you to include what you may have considered minutiae in your publication manuscript, so having a detailed draft allows you to pull the information without having to re-request the notes from Medical Records.

9.2.2 Patient consent

This is a key requirement for most reputable publishers, and many will have their own forms that will need to be completed and have the patient's signature as a mark of his or her consent. This often means that you have to make an early decision regarding to which organisation you are going to submit your article. If you don't, we would suggest using a generic non-branded consent form.

We advise getting consent early – ideally while the patient is still an inpatient (if he or she does become an inpatient) – for various reasons, not limited to but including the fact that you don't want to spend lots of time writing a full case report only to be denied permission to publish it by the patient, but also, patients often have useful insights into their condition and presentation, with some publishers providing a section for a statement from the patient in the final publication.

If you don't manage to get the consent while the patient is an inpatient, don't be embarrassed to telephone the patient and ask for his or her consent. You can then post a consent form with a stamped envelope in which to return the signed form. Where a patient is deceased, publishers will often accept the next of kin's consent, which can be obtained in a sensitive way after a reasonable period of mourning has elapsed – please be sensitive.

Case Study 9.2 Consent for case reports

The patient discussed in our case report 'Thoracic Oesophageal Cancer as a Cause of Stridor: A Literature Review' [1] was too unwell for us to approach regarding consent during her inpatient stay in our unit and, unfortunately, passed away 2 months later. Our team felt this was an important presentation whose associated literature review could inform the management of future patients; therefore, after a sufficient period of waiting, we contacted the patient's next of kin, who approved of the article's educational objectives. We sent them a consent form via post with a stamped envelope, which they promptly returned signed, and we proceeded to write and publish the article.

Chapter 9

9.2.3 Images

Images are a crucial part of case reports – they are proof of your diagnosis, and readers particularly enjoy looking at radiological scans and identifying abnormalities themselves. It is rare to find a published case report in a respectable journal that does not feature images of one type or another. These images can be clinical, radiological, or histological.

9.2.3.1 Clinical photographs

Clinical photographs can be obtained in cooperation with your hospital's Medical Illustration department where there is time to send the patient for photography, as this is a professional service that will ensure high-quality images. However, where there is no time to send the patient to Medical Illustration, e.g. a medical emergency, and the patient gives his or her consent, photographs can be taken with one's high-resolution camera, provided they are kept in a secure location, e.g. hospital computer hard drive. Devices such as endoscopic video monitors have the facility to photograph and store images in clinic or intraoperatively – such images are an elegant way of showing examination findings.

9.2.3.2 Radiological studies

Radiological studies are essential when presenting your case, and where the radiologist has not marked the abnormality and you are not sure, we strongly advise discussing and collaborating with a radiologist to obtain the best image possible. Many individuals in specialist practice are able to interpret radiological studies pertinent to their specialty, thus it will be very embarrassing for you to submit a radiological imaging showing one thing that you've labelled as another – such faux pas won't get past the peer review process of a reputable journal and will undermine you in the eyes of the reviewers.

9.2.3.3 Histology slides

Histopathological images are also an interesting addition to a case report. Although they may not be as much of a necessity as a radiological image, particularly given that they are not as widely well interpreted by the majority of clinicians, they can illustrate a disease process in a unique way. We recommend speaking to a pathologist early, as they may require time to prepare the slides to a standard suitable for publication. This is especially important if a long period of time has elapsed from when they reported the results, as the slides may have been put into a storage facility.

9.2.4 Data protection

Please ensure you make every attempt to guarantee that the information you write is anonymised. Most countries, especially in the European Union, have strict data protection laws, which are based on protecting an individual's data. It's important to make sure you remove any names, addresses, dates of birth, and other patient identifiable information from your draft and from any images you may use.

Do not keep anything that might contain patient identifiable information on your own personal devices. This ensures you never fall afoul of your employer or the law. You can, of course, continue to work on completely anonymised drafts on your personal devices.

9.3 Writing the case report

As a comprehensive treatment of writing a paper is given in Chapter 7 of this book, this chapter will only focus on the practicalities of the topic as it relates to writing up a case report.

At this point, it is prudent to have decided on the journal to which you are going to submit. Most journals have guidelines on the format in which they want the case to be presented, and some even have a template in which you simply enter the relevant information. Also note any word limits given by the journal and ensure you stick to them. Most reputable journals have incorporated the CARE (CAse REport) Checklist into their submissions process or advise you to ensure your report meets these guidelines. These guidelines are the current international consensus on how to present a case report, and the checklist can be found on the CARE website – http://www. care-statement.org.

We have summarised it into the following components, which can be used to fill the checklist: introduction, case, discussion, and conclusion.

We do not discuss patient perspective in detail, as it is not an essential requirement, and some patients find it cumbersome to be asked to write a section for a scientific journal. However, we would encourage you to ask the patient if he or she would like to give a perspective on the case. It is prudent to do this during the consent phase, as well as after you have written the case, providing the patient with a final copy of what you wish to publish. This is because, after a period of recovery and reflecting on what you have written, the patient may be willing to write about his or her perspective or at least offer you feedback on your article.

9.3.1 Introduction

Aim to introduce your topic in a succinct manner, giving background information on the condition but not discussing your specific patient. You may want to include epidemiological information as well as any information that relates to the angle at which you are approaching the topic.

Chapter 9

Case Study 9.3 Introduction

In our previously mentioned case report [1], the focus was on how rare stridor was as an initial presentation for oesophageal cancer. Therefore, the introduction to the article describes the condition and then references a large study by the American College of Surgeons where they do not even list stridor as a symptom, to show how unusual it is to see such a presentation.

Similarly, in the our case series – 'Unusual Childhood Presentations of Abdominal non-Hodgkin's Lymphoma' [2] – background on lymphoma is given, but the discussion is steered quickly to presentations of this disease and why specifically abdominal non-Hodgkin's lymphoma is of interest – namely, that it can present like an acute surgical abdomen and be difficult to differentiate from this condition.

9.3.2 Case presentation

We recommend presenting the case as one would during a long case at university or a new patient to his or her seniors on a ward round. This involves stating some pertinent background initially, giving an account of the presenting complaint and its history, followed by associated symptoms, then investigations and diagnosis. This is a format with which many are familiar and comfortable in terms of presenting, and one that many readers are used to hearing in their daily practice – it therefore gives you the advantage of readability and familiarity.

Case Study 9.4 The case presentation

In the case report 'Re-expansion Pulmonary Oedema: A Novel Therapeutic Option', the first case begins:

> A 68-year-old woman, with a background of metastatic breast cancer, type-2 diabetes mellitus, and hypercholesterolaemia, presented with a 1-week history of dyspnoea, palpitations, and presyncope when mobilising. She also reported of a dry cough and had recently finished a course of palliative capecitabine chemotherapy. She lived with her family and was largely independent. She was a non-smoker. A chest x-ray demonstrated a large left-sided pleural effusion.

This layout demonstrates an easy to read, familiar format in which you can include pertinent clinical information whilst maintaining the reader's attention. This does take time to learn effectively, and one may not be at a sufficient level of medical education to be regularly presenting patients or in a healthcare discipline where it is not a common occurrence, therefore, we recommend involving your seniors and other members of the multidisciplinary team and having them read and provide feedback. This is an essential part of the process because it allows you to learn directly from those around you who have experience in this area.

9.3.3 Discussion

Use this section to discuss the overall case – from the patient presentation, to assessment and treatment, and even to the outcome. You can comment on all of these in the discussion section, including explaining your team's rationale for any treatment decisions. You should also use this section to discuss where your case report fits within the body of medical literature. It is an opportunity to present your findings in comparison with what has already been written. In order to do this, you need to perform a literature review – the specifics of which are discussed in Chapter 3. As you conduct your literature review, consider how each article you are reading relates to your own article and what would be important for readers to know about the subject.

It may help to consider the following questions:

- Why did I write this case report?
- What is unique or peculiar about the case?
- What is the current evidence surrounding the topic about which I am writing?
- What are the key learning points for people's practice?

Frame the answers to these questions in logical prose for your discussion section. It's important to keep a structure to your discussion – dealing with one subject at a time and linking it either to the overall topic or the next subject. If this is not doable, don't hesitate to break it down into sections that make it easier for you to discuss the case.

Case Study 9.5 Discussion

The 'Discussion' section for our case report 'Concomitant AIDS Cholangiopathy and Fanconi Syndrome as Complications of HIV in a Single Patient' [3] is split into two sections, the first section discussing Fanconi syndrome and the second focusing on AIDS cholangiopathy. This allowed for both important topics to be discussed adequately, without any confusion for the reader.

9.3.4 Conclusion

This is a short summary of your article. You can mention your case in one line and what it shows, but ensure to focus on the learning points and what you want the reader to take away from your article. An additional point may be to consider what, if any, further research could be conducted into the topic, in order to answer any questions you or others have raised.

Case Study 9.6 Conclusion

In our case series on non-Hodgkin's lymphoma [2], we conclude that the disease can have a variety of clinical presentations. We highlight this as the main learning point of the case series and implore paediatricians to keep this important diagnosis in the differential when caring for children with abdominal pain.

Chapter 9

References

1. Maweni, R.M., Manikavasagar, V., Sunderland, N., and Chaudhry, S. (2018). Thoracic oesophageal cancer as a cause of stridor: a literature review. *BMJ Case Rep.* **2018**: bcr-2018-224872. https://www.ncbi.nlm.nih.gov/pubmed/29844036.
2. Foley, R.W., Aworanti, O.M., Gorman, L. et al. (2016). Unusual childhood presentations of abdominal non-Hodgkin's lymphoma. *Pediatr. Int.* **58**: 304–307. https://www.ncbi.nlm.nih.gov/pubmed/26670157.
3. Maweni, R., Kallampallil, J., Leong, S., and Akunuri, S. (2017). Concomitant AIDS cholangiopathy and Fanconi syndrome as complications of HIV in a single patient. *BMJ Case Rep.* **2017**: bcr-2017-222333. https://www.ncbi.nlm.nih.gov/pubmed/29167218.

Chapter 10 **Basic laboratory research**

10.1 Introduction to laboratory research and translational research

Underlying nearly every treatment you deliver in your profession is years and years of basic research. This basic research often takes place inside the laboratory as opposed to the clinic, and it is important to understand how this kind of research takes place and why you might want to get involved in it.

Basic research, also sometimes called wet lab research or pre-clinical research depending on the setting, is a phase of research that takes place in the laboratory before any involvement of human subjects and often involves the use of tissue samples, cell lines, and model organisms such as mice and flies. This is a crucial phase of research that helps to establish therapeutic targets, efficacy, safety profiles, and the overall viability of new therapeutic methods before they are tested on humans.

In recent years, this process of moving a therapeutic target from the pre-clinical phase to the clinical phase has grown progressively more difficult as researchers and clinicians alike struggle to come to grips with complex diseases, especially those associated with ageing like cancer and neurodegenerative diseases. This, alongside the uptick in massive datasets from large genomic and proteomic studies, has meant that new approaches are needed to effectively tackle this problem.

As such, the promotion of the concept of translational or 'bench to bedside' research has grown significantly. Translational research is a way of improving the connection between pre-clinical and clinical research in order to improve the efficiency of transitioning therapeutics from the lab, into clinical practice and to the bedside.

How to Succeed in Medical Research: A Practical Guide, First Edition.
Robert Foley, Robert Maweni, Shahram Shirazi, and Hussein Jaafar.
© 2021 John Wiley & Sons Ltd. Published 2021 by John Wiley & Sons Ltd.
Companion website: www.wiley.com/go/foley/succeed

10.2 Basic research versus clinical research

The majority of people reading this book are likely to be familiar with the setting, demands, and day-to-day activities of researchers in the clinical field. A good way to introduce you to basic research is to compare and contrast these two disciplines. The first comparison is of course the scope of the research. By that I mean the differences in what is being researched and the immediate impact of discoveries made in that scope.

A major discovery made in basic research may take many years or even decades to bear fruit in the day-to-day lives of ordinary people in the community, but the range of people it may impact can be far greater. A major clinical discovery could be applicable and transferable to the treatment phase in far less time, but that discovery is also likely to be limited in its range of applicability.

This makes sense when we understand that basic researchers are often studying phenomena and processes that are very fundamental to the operation of a cell, bacteria, virus, or plant, without too much consideration (at least initially) as to how this might be affecting higher-order processes. This type of research is often very slow and complicated to carry out. For example, a researcher might be studying a new protein involved in the process of autophagy in the model organism *Saccharomyces cerevisiae* (baker's yeast). Now of course any discovery made with this model organism would have to first be confirmed in mammalian (at least mice if not human) cells before any sort of therapeutic outcome could be devised. It may be that this protein does not even exist in mammalian cells, and if it does it may have a completely different function. However, if this protein and process is in fact conserved between the model organism and human cells, then it is likely to be of great importance to the functioning of our cells and could birth many new therapeutic developments.

Clinical researchers, on the other hand, usually start working with mammalian cells from the onset and often are studying well-understood proteins, genes, or processes in a more direct manner, testing the response of these to chemicals, drugs, gene manipulation, harsh environments, etc. Usually the outcome of such experiments, if successful, would be directed at a single disease or therapeutic outcome.

Practically speaking, the kinds of experiments you will do also differ in basic vs clinical research. One striking difference is the involvement of patients and the individual vs teamwork environment. Basic researchers are very unlikely to work with patients unless it is in the context of using patient cells or tissues. Furthermore, basic researchers generally do not work with colleagues on a daily basis, at least not for the purposes of carrying out experiments. Meetings, discussions, and mentoring will naturally take place, but the day-to-day planning and handling of experiments is often left to the individual researcher to do. Clinical researchers, on the other hand, are generally more team-oriented. The nature of their experiments often necessitates close collaboration and regular interaction with both fellow researchers and patients.

10.3 Laboratory hierarchy

Another major difference is the hierarchy of the lab in a basic vs clinical setting. Or perhaps more accurately, the difference in hierarchy in a university or dedicated research institute laboratory vs in a hospital setting. In a university or dedicated research institute, the hierarchy is as follows in descending seniority:

- Principal investigator (PI: usually but not always a professor).
- Postdoctoral researcher (aka a postdoc; a researcher who has already finished his or her PhD).
- PhD candidate.
- Master's student.
- Bachelor's student or a research elective student.

The PI in turn would report to the head of his or her department but is generally autonomous in the handling of the lab and students. Depending on the size and specific organisation of the lab, you may find yourself under the supervision of a late-stage PhD candidate, a postdoc, or even the PIs themselves.

In the clinical setting, the hierarchy may not be so clearly defined. You may be working independently on a research project, under the supervision of your mentor. In this case your project will be operating outside the normal clinical team's structure, although it is important to recognise that you may be working alongside colleagues in their clinical roles when you are collecting data or presenting your results at a departmental meeting. In the hospital, there may be a research nurse or assistant who operates from the hospital and may be a great source of help for you.

In large academic centres worldwide, often clinical research and laboratory research co-exist side by side, sometimes in the same building. You may find yourself straddling both worlds, especially if your supervisor is an active doctor in a clinical speciality and also runs his or her own research lab. Being aware of the hierarchy of a lab, therefore, will come in handy, even if you are not carrying out basic research yourself. Try to get to know colleagues who are working under your supervisor in basic science research. Perhaps they

Chapter 10

need some help, which could be a fantastic opportunity for you to gain experience in lab research!

10.4 Day to day of working in the lab

The day-to-day working life in the lab varies significantly depending on which day of the week it is and what kind of lab you are in, but there are certain elements that are consistent throughout.

10.4.1 Documentation

Documentation is an invaluable part of working in the lab. This primarily takes the form of a lab book. The lab book is either a physical or increasingly digital log in which you note the details of your daily experiments, their outcomes, and the manner in which they were conducted. You will constantly need to refer back to your lab book, and researchers who omit details or daily logs in their books will do so at their own peril! Too often a detail that seemed unimportant at the time will suddenly be critical to figuring out why your experiment didn't work 3 months down the line. One can never be too sure, and an extra 5 minutes spent writing the precise parameters of your experiment can save many headache-filled days later on.

10.4.2 Lab meetings

Another regular aspect is the lab meeting. These are usually weekly meetings in which some or all members of your lab group will gather to discuss the latest results from experiments, strategies for projects, publication prospects, and schedules and offer advice and support to one another. The latter can be especially important when issues arise during your experiments. It is an important time for assessing how your experiments are progressing and to gain insights and practical advice from more senior or experienced lab members. It's also good practise for your presentation skills, which you can hone for use at conferences or scientific retreats.

10.4.3 Lab upkeep

Depending on the size of your lab and whether or not your supervisor employs technical assistants, another common duty will be the cleaning and upkeep of equipment, reagents, and chemical and biological stocks. This requires detailed knowledge of the recipes, volumes, temperatures, pH, and safety and hazard warnings of your stocks or equipment and is vital to ensuring that when something is needed for an experiment, it is ready to go and not in need of cleaning, restocking, or calibration!

10.4.4 Reading

The final daily task you will likely find yourself engaging in is reading. Whether it is looking up papers to find a protocol you wish to do or reading a review to try and make sense of your latest results, reading takes up a significant portion of your time. Most basic research involves long periods of waiting. This can be because your experiment is incubating, your cells are growing, your code is compiling, or your polymerase chain reaction (PCR) is cycling. In these long stretches, often the best thing to do is read. It would be advisable to take this time to organise your readings properly and systematically. One way to do this is by using a paper and citation management tool, as mentioned in Chapter 3, such as Zotero, Endnote, or Mendeley. Every time you read a paper that contains some useful or interesting information, you can save that paper to your paper management programme of choice and leave notes or highlight the relevant points of interest. Done properly and from the beginning of your project, you can have a treasure trove of well-curated and documented sources that will form the core of future papers or dissertations you write.

Case Study 10.1 Troubleshooting experiments

Here I will describe an experiment that you may perform in a basic research lab. In doing so, I hope you will gain an insight into the way different experimental techniques can combine to achieve a result in your topic of interest. I will explain the basic principles of these techniques as I go along. These will include microscopy, DNA/plasmid isolation, primer design, PCR, and cell culturing.

Let's suppose I have a newly discovered protein – let's call it protein X – that I am interested in investigating. I want to investigate this protein using the model organism *S. cerevisiae* (baker's yeast), a very popular organism to use for basic molecular biology research. One of the first things you can do to uncover a potential aspect of protein X is to find out where in the cell it is located. The location of the protein in the cell can provide strong hints as to its function, whether it's at the nucleus, cell wall, mitochondria, etc. There are several ways you could do this, but one common method is to look at the protein microscopically.

Most individual proteins are too small and too indistinct to observe directly under a microscope. So in order to detect your protein microscopically, you can attach what is known as a fluorescent protein to it. Probably the most popular of the fluorescent proteins is green fluorescent protein (GFP). Fluorescent proteins are proteins that when exposed to particular wavelengths of light will fluoresce with a coloured light, which can be detected using a

Chapter 10

confocal microscope. Therefore, if you attach a GFP to your protein of interest, when this new fusion protein is exposed to light of the correct wavelength, you will see a green fluorescence under the microscope, revealing the location of your protein of interest within the cell.

To attach GFP to protein X, we need to use something called a plasmid. A plasmid is a circular type of DNA commonly used by bacteria and other microorganisms to express their constitutive proteins. Nowadays these plasmids are easy for researchers to manipulate genetically and so are often used to express proteins of interest in model organisms such as bacteria and yeast cells. Typically your lab will have stocks of bacteria that contain a plasmid expressing various different proteins, including fluorescent proteins like GFP. You can take a sample of bacteria that contains a plasmid expressing GFP and culture the bacteria until you have a large enough quantity to use experimentally. You can then harvest these bacterial cells and isolate the GFP containing plasmids from them. Once this is done, you can carry out a PCR, which will allow you to extract specifically the GFP sequence from the plasmid. When you conduct this PCR, you also take care to design the DNA primers (short strands of DNA that initiate the PCR reaction), so that they contain overhangs (basically extra bits of DNA) that are specific for your protein of interest. This means when the GFP sequence undergoes the PCR, it will have on either side of it an overhang that matches to the sequence of our protein of interest. This will be important later when inserting the GFP sequence next to the sequence of protein X.

This GFP sequence can then be inserted just before the beginning of proteins X's sequence on the relevant chromosomes in your yeast cells. This is done via a technique called homologous recombination, which involves culturing your yeast cells in a mixture with your GFP sequence, briefly opening the cell walls of yeast via heat shock, which then allows the GFP sequence to get inside the cells. By random chance the overhangs on our GFP sequence, which again are designed to match the sequence at the beginning of protein X, will cause the entire GFP sequence to be inserted into the chromosomal DNA of our yeast cells. The odds of this happening are quite low, but given that we are culturing millions of cells at a time, they are high enough to make the technique reliable. Now since the GFP sequence and protein X's sequence are side by side on the chromosome, the two proteins will be expressed together as fusion protein! Looking at this new fusion protein under a confocal microscope will now allow you to visualise the location of protein X.

10.5 How to choose your lab

In this chapter, we have discussed a lot about what working in a lab is like and what you can expect if you get involved in it. So what are some things to look out for when you search for a lab?

Working in the lab requires a particular mindset. While the work can be rewarding, as you solve complex puzzles and questions, leading investigations at the edge of known science, it is also very challenging, isolating, and frustrating work. The difficulties and rewards of doing lab research in general are discussed in detail in Chapter 11, in Case Study 11.5, 'Undertaking a PhD'. This is applicable also to research carried out as part of a master's or other programme. If you are set on pursuing research in a lab, there are three major areas you should consider.

Firstly, make sure to choose a topic you are genuinely interested in. In a way, all research can be fascinating if you have a naturally curious disposition. After all, most basic research labs are fundamentally trying to answer the same broad questions. What does this protein do? How can we manipulate this biological process? How does this external condition affect this gene expression? The only differences in the questions asked are the specific field it's being asked in, whether that is neuroscience, cancer genetics, or microbiology. Ultimately, though, it is still important to choose a lab you feel is carrying out research you are motivated to participate in. This above all else can help drive your work and will help sustain you through difficult periods. Consider how the topic you choose can fit with your existing knowledge or studies. Alternatively, you might want to branch out and pick a subject that is completely outside of your realm of expertise just because there is something about it that excites you or that you feel might help make your knowledge set more rounded.

Secondly, choosing a good supervisor is critical but also very tricky to do. Typically you may only get to have a handful of relatively brief discussions with your prospective supervisor before you have to make a decision on joining his or her lab. Therefore, it is incredibly important to ask key questions during this time that will help you determine if you will receive the kind and level of supervision and guidance you expect. Some questions you might like to ask are:

- Who will be my direct supervisor? The lab head, a postdoctoral researcher, or a PhD student?
- How many people are in the lab? How much daily or weekly contact can I expect from the supervisor?

- What is his or her supervising style?
- How often has the lab published? At least yearly is a good rule of thumb for a decent lab, not including review papers or similar.
- How often are lab meetings held?
- What are the expectations of the supervisor? How many hours a week should I be working? What kind of end result is the supervisor expecting – an entire paper, or just some additional insights or data?

In these discussions, it would be pertinent at this point to also highlight to your prospective supervisor your expectations. You should also set up some monthly/yearly goals for the project with a system to regularly update these as plans change. Think about the relationship you want to have with your prospective supervisor. Do you want the person to be very hands-on in guidance and help, or do you prefer a hands-off approach? Should you set up a schedule for regular meetings to re-assess the project and the dynamic between student and supervisor? Are you willing to work outside of contracted or expected hours? Is this what the supervisor expects of you? In too many cases, research is frustrated by poor communication between the involved parties. Make sure to be as open and honest about your needs, expectations, and requirements before and throughout the time you spend in research.

Thirdly, ensure you have a clear idea of how doing research will advance your own personal and professional progression. Perhaps there are particular skills you want to learn, such as data analysis, handling and use of specialised equipment, etc. Perhaps you want to become an expert in a specific topic that interests you or to supplement your medical knowledge. Perhaps you want to bolster your career prospects. All of these are valid reasons in and of themselves, and it's important to understand your own inspirations for doing research. Doing so will help you to choose a lab that best reflects your motivations and allow you to work towards those goals more effectively.

Chapter 11 **Expanding your horizons in research**

There are a number of avenues within research to further your career, ranging from research electives to PhD studies. The route you take will depend on a number of personal factors, including your ability to move homes, afford to undertake a research degree, or obtain funding. It is important to consider the time implications that are necessary when applying for higher training, such as a master's degree, and the potential impact on income if you are unable to work during this time. Most importantly, you must decide whether or not an elective or further research degree fits in with your career aspirations.

11.1 Research elective

Research electives offer the opportunity to undertake a shorter period of research experience, in the region of 4–12 weeks. These can be done both in your home country or abroad. They may also be an excellent opportunity to visit a foreign institution and work alongside researchers who are experts in their field. Research teams are often very happy to take on students for an elective, as although there may be a period of training, often the relationship is symbiotic, with the student gaining valuable experience but also helping to produce results for the team. The best method to undertake a research elective is to visit the website of a hospital or university and see what is available. Or, if you know of a research topic you are very interested in, find out who are the important researchers in that field and get in contact with them. Although research electives are generally for students, if you are working you may be able to complete a research observership instead and still gain this valuable experience.

How to Succeed in Medical Research: A Practical Guide, First Edition.
Robert Foley, Robert Maweni, Shahram Shirazi, and Hussein Jaafar.
© 2021 John Wiley & Sons Ltd. Published 2021 by John Wiley & Sons Ltd.
Companion website: www.wiley.com/go/foley/succeed

Case Study 11.1 Neurological research elective

I attended the Irish Neurological Association meeting, and the keynote speaker was a research professor at Johns Hopkins Hospital in Baltimore, Maryland. His research interest was multiple sclerosis, and he delivered an excellent talk at the conference. I was very impressed, and although I had very little experience in neurological research, I thought this was a brilliant opportunity for a research elective. I did some information collecting online and found that research electives at Johns Hopkins were not very expensive; although a clinical elective (in neurology, for example) would cost thousands of dollars, a research elective was only $300. This would be affordable for me, and so I got in touch with the professor with the following email:

***

Dear Professor. . .,

I recently attended your lecture at the Irish Neurological Association meeting. I found it incredibly interesting, and despite your overarching clinical spin on the talk I found the basic science portions the most compelling.

I am a final year medical student at University College Dublin and if acceptable I would love to visit your institution. I would like to perform a research elective and join your research team, for example at weekly lab meetings, journal club etc., but also potentially join you in the outpatient clinic setting to gain some experience of patient management.

I believe I'd stand to learn an awful lot from such an experience and if you agree and would like to have me I'd be delighted to begin an application through the School of Medicine.

Thank you for your time.

Kind regards,

***

I received a favourable response and carried out a 4-week research elective. It was a fantastic experience to work with a fantastic research team and to experience a different healthcare system.

11.2 Intercalated research degree

An intercalated degree is an excellent opportunity to gain some research experience during your undergraduate degree. In some cases an intercalated degree is a built-in portion of the degree that everyone undertakes, in other cases you must attempt to organise this for yourself. Often funding is available for this through a competitive process. If so, this is a wonderful opportunity and will give you time to carry out full-time research, which will allow you to fully engage with a project rather than having to do so in small chunks. This will also give you the chance to see if a research career is for you, offering you a trial period as a full-time researcher.

Case Study 11.2 Intercalated master of science

Following on from a summer period of research during my medical training (as mentioned in Chapter 1), I then applied for an intercalated MSc scholarship from my university. The process consisted of an application form, in which I was asked to outline my research interests and my previous experience in research, provide my grades in medical school thus far, and give a personal statement. The next stage of the process was an interview, in which I gave a 15-minute presentation on my research proposal, followed by a 15-minute period of questions. I also decided to print off my research proposal for the panel of interviewers before my presentation. I also printed off my CV and my academic transcript for the interviewers to look through if they wished. I gave this to each interviewer in a binder, to make it all look neat and professional. I was successful at the interview and awarded a scholarship for my MSc.

11.3 Postgraduate diplomas/certificates

These qualifications generally require a year or 2 of full-time or part-time education. These can be undertaken in a huge variety of subjects and are an excellent chance to expand your knowledge. However, these courses can be expensive if you don't obtain funding, so be sure this is what you would like to pursue before applying.

Chapter 11

Case Study 11.3 Graduate certificate in mathematics and statistics

Following on from my MSc, in which I began to learn some statistics and analyse data, I was keen to learn more. I applied for a part-time graduate certificate in statistics from the University of Sheffield. I began by researching which universities in the UK offered part-time courses in statistics, and I believed the course in Sheffield was the most suited to my needs. As I was working full time as a doctor, many of the courses were not suitable for me because I needed to be present for classes during the week. This was not realistic for me as I would not be able to attend regularly. However, the course I was applying to offered me the opportunity to complete my weekly modules and assignments at any time, which was the flexibility I needed to go along with a shift pattern job. I decided to go down this route, as I knew it was an excellent opportunity for me to build upon my statistical knowledge and make the best use of my time. This qualification allowed me to gain a deeper understanding of how to carry out well-designed research studies and learn new methods of data analysis.

11.4 Postgraduate degree

A master's degree or PhD can be undertaken as a postgraduate, following completion of your undergraduate degree. There are a huge variety of subjects that can be studied during these degrees. When it comes to a master's degree, you can decide to undertake a period of study that is more focused on your future career interests, as can be seen from the next case study. A PhD is a very specialised research degree in which you will focus on a very narrow field of study; before you undertake a PhD you are likely to have spent a lot of previous time researching your PhD topic. This is the highest qualification that can be undertaken and takes a period of 3–5 years to complete. Undertaking a PhD is an opportunity to become an expert in your field of research, and this can be achieved in a number of ways; however, a common route to a PhD is through laboratory research.

Chapter 11

Case Study 11.4 Master's in surgery

Whilst working as a junior doctor, I had decided on a career in surgery. I was also interested in furthering my understanding of research, and so a part-time master's in surgery (MCh) was an excellent option for me. Over the course of 2 years, I carried out regular modules in surgical research, which covered research design, research methods, biostatistics, surgical education, and human factors in surgery. The degree then culminated in an original research project and thesis submission. The ability to study for this MCh part time over 2 years allowed me to learn whilst working as a surgical trainee. And importantly, studying for a master's degree that was tailored to surgery was a brilliant opportunity to learn skills that would be useful in my future career.

Case Study 11.5 Undertaking a PhD

Perhaps the most demanding academic route is the PhD. This is usually a 3- to 5-year, full-time undertaking in which the entirety of your time is dedicated to a single topic. Not to be pursed lightly, one must consider carefully his or her interest in a topic as well as the potential pitfalls and disadvantages.

Most major universities will have PhD programmes in various topics. Applications to one of these programmes can vary. One common type of application you will find is a general application to a PhD programme within a department covering a broad topic, say neuroscience. These types of applications will involve panel interviews and tours of the facilities and different labs within a department. If you are successful in getting the offer of a position in the programme, you will usually be assigned a specific project afterwards. Sometimes this means spending the first year of the PhD doing rotations in different labs within the department you applied to, before settling on a project you like at the end of the rotations. Another way you can apply to a PhD is by finding individual programmes offered by a lab directly. In contrast to the more general applications, this process will involve directly speaking to the head of the lab you applied to and interviewing with just the lab head and/or your prospective supervisor/mentor.

First I'll talk about the advantages and attractive aspects of doing a PhD. First and perhaps foremost for a lot of people, it is simply the best and really the only way to pursue a long-term career in traditional academia. If you wish to be a professor at a university or to lead your own research lab, you need to be an expert in your field, and a PhD is often a necessity to that end. Therefore, if your passion truly is conducting research and being at the cutting edge of scientific discovery, a PhD is certainly something you should consider.

Beyond this a PhD is actually a generally excellent training programme that can give you experience in a wide variety of skills and techniques that you can use in all aspects of your professional career. Long-term strategic planning, troubleshooting, public speaking, writing, understanding and synthesising complex topics, unique and varied technical experience (microscopy, stem cell culturing, 3D modelling, etc.) – these are just some of the areas of expertise you will get unmatched training in. All of these can benefit you long after the PhD is over, even if you don't stay in academia. PhD graduates are often highly sought after precisely for the high degree of skilled training they have received.

You will also have the possibility of accessing some of the best equipment and working with some of the brightest minds in the world today. Institutes that have PhD research programmes often attract the most respected and advanced researchers. It is an opportunity to interact and gain knowledge and experience from the best of the best.

Now to talk about the downsides to a PhD, and as you will likely have heard, there are many, which is why it is strongly advised to think carefully before embarking on this path. A PhD is gruelling, frustrating, regularly unrewarding work. You will work long hours; 12 hour days plus weekends is common, especially during crunch times. Financially speaking, PhDs are not very well compensated for the hours worked or the degree of technical or theoretical knowledge required to do their work. Your experience in the lab can also be highly dependent on your supervisor and lab colleagues. Having a good supervisor can make the PhD experience manageable. On the other hand, a bad supervisor can make your experience much more difficult. You will spend countless days or weeks on a single experiment that won't work no matter what you try, and it can be nearly impossible to figure out why due to the number of variables involved. Sometimes you simply have to give up on an experiment and move on even after spending many agonising hours on it. It's not uncommon to completely abandon your project and switch to another one halfway through your PhD. If all of this sounds incredibly frustrating, that's because it is, and you need to be prepared to deal with significant amounts of mental and physical stress if you are to complete your PhD.

The other side of this is that when you emerge out the other side of your PhD, you will likely be incredibly well prepared for anything that your future professional career throws at you. Be sure to speak to as many people as you can prior to embarking on a PhD application, both those students studying for a PhD and those who have already completed the degree.

Chapter 11

Chapter 12 **Teaching**

12.1 How to get involved in teaching

Teaching can be one of the most enjoyable aspects of being a healthcare professional – there is great joy to be had from facilitating or actively participating in the education of others, be they your contemporaries or other members of the multidisciplinary team. However, it can also be a daunting task. We recommend that you think of it as an opportunity to share your experiences and expertise. Remember that at whatever level you are and in whatever discipline you are, you have knowledge, skills, and attitudes from which someone else can learn. There are, therefore, myriad opportunities for you to use these and get involved in teaching; however, you often need to seek them out. For this purpose, it is useful to think of teaching as formal or informal.

Formal teaching is part of a structured programme with a curriculum and externally agreed, prespecified objectives run by an organisation like a university or hospital. Examples of this include being a university anatomy demonstrator. This is a post recognised by the university, often paid, where the demonstrator supervises cadaveric dissection sessions as well as teaching anatomy through already prosected cadaveric specimens.

With Informal teaching, however, there is no structured programme or prespecified curriculum by an organisation. It is often done to fit the needs of the learners and often depends on the goodwill of ordinary people who can provide the knowledge. An example of this is bedside teaching. This often takes place in teaching hospitals, in which willing teachers – e.g. a senior student or junior doctor or even retired consultant – make themselves available to a group of students to see a patient who is currently in the hospital and discuss this patient's condition. This can include a discussion of history taking, examination findings, investigations for a particular condition, as well as the management of said condition. The teachers are not paid by the

How to Succeed in Medical Research: A Practical Guide, First Edition.
Robert Foley, Robert Maweni, Shahram Shirazi, and Hussein Jaafar.
© 2021 John Wiley & Sons Ltd. Published 2021 by John Wiley & Sons Ltd.
Companion website: www.wiley.com/go/foley/succeed

university for the express purpose of delivering this teaching, nor are they keeping to a university-specific curriculum – often they are teaching practical aspects that will be useful in practice and in practical examinations.

12.2 Teaching as an undergraduate student

University can seem like a difficult place at which to get involved in teaching. There are other important factors such as your level of knowledge, level of confidence, and balancing studying and your personal life. There may also be a relative paucity of opportunities for students to be teachers. However, as with most things, if you seek out the opportunities, you will find them. We recommend speaking directly to the faculty as a first point. This might be a lecturer in a subject you're interested in, or even the dean of your programme. It is often easier to make an appointment and do it in person; however, an email can do the trick just as well.

Simply introduce yourself, state that you have an interest in teaching, and ask if the person has, or knows of, any opportunities available for a student to teach. If you are a relatively senior student, you may even suggest roles you have seen other students undertake, such as anatomy demonstrations or performing tutorials.

If you are very early in your studies, for example, as a first- or second-year undergraduate, it may be prudent to build up your teaching experience by taking part in tutoring and mentoring of secondary school students and more junior students in your discipline. Such experience will help to give you a competitive edge when applying for teaching roles at the undergraduate level, as they show your experience and commitment to teaching. These

> **Case Study 12.1 University teaching – the early years**
> During my first year in medical school, I joined my university's Higher Education Access Route (HEAR) tutoring programme. In this programme I tutored final-year secondary school/high school students in biology, with a particular focus on examination preparation. This was a formal post, recognised and paid by the university, which was very useful on my CV going forward as well as a much-needed source of income for a student!
>
> I also then took the opportunity as a second-year medical student to mentor the new first-year students, and whilst this was not a paid position, it still provided valuable experience and was a useful addition to an otherwise barren CV. This, again, was an informal role, but it allowed me to use the skills and knowledge I had gained in the previous year to make a difference for the students I was mentoring.

> **Case Study 12.2 University teaching – the later years**
>
> During my senior years in medical school, I reached out to the head of anatomy and the neuroanatomy lead at my university to discuss potential teaching opportunities. I met with both individuals after introducing myself by email; however, I was not given the opportunity straight away. I persisted with keeping in touch, and just before the start of a new semester, I was given a role as an anatomy tutor for the neurology module. I was delighted with this, as neurology was my favourite topic in medical school. I began to give weekly tutorials and also functioned as a demonstrator during the dissection practicals for the second-year medical students.
>
> From this initial teaching opportunity grew many more, and because the professor came to know me, I was offered teaching opportunities in a number of other courses in the medical school. I also gave tutorials in healthcare informatics and was a demonstrator for the computer-assisted laboratory sessions on radiology. Although I was still a medical student at this time, I had completed the modules I was teaching a couple of years earlier, and so with some extra preparation time, I was able to effectively teach the learning objectives for each session.

opportunities can be sought by reaching out to the admissions/access teams, who may run programmes tutoring secondary school students in subjects you have previously performed well in. Mentoring opportunities can be sought by reaching out to the appropriate dean for first-year undergraduates.

12.3 Teaching as a postgraduate student

The opportunity to get involved in teaching is often associated with postgraduate studies, such as a master's degree, which may involve taking an extra year to carry out a research project. Teaching can be carried out alongside your degree – allowing you to grow your research and teaching portfolios at the same time. Some degrees may be associated with a summer research project, which can be just as fruitful, and will, at the very least, allow you to build useful networks for research and teaching in the future.

Often, full-time postgraduate courses offer students the opportunity to undertake teaching as a part of the formal programme. If you are already undertaking a postgraduate degree or PhD and don't have formal teaching sessions built into your programme, we strongly encourage you to discuss the possibilities with your supervisor and ask, where your schedule allows, to gain some teaching experience.

Chapter 12

Case Study 12.3 Teaching as a postgraduate

During my MSc studies, I was a supervisor for a final-year BSc student (biomedical health and life science) during his 4-month research placement, which culminates in a thesis submission. I was offered the position and at first I thought it would be quite daunting. The thesis forms one-half of each student's final-year credits, and so it is clearly incredibly important to each student's degree. I did, however, take on the role.

I spoke to the head of my lab about the best way to go about supervising my new student, and together we came up with a defined research project for his rotation. I then oversaw my student's progress on a day-to-day basis, making sure everything was still going on schedule and being on hand to help with any issues as they arose. We also scheduled a more formal weekly meeting to make sure his progress was on track. Although quite difficult at times to be responsible for another student, and of course responsible for my own research at the same time, I still found this to be an important learning experience. It also allowed me to see the reverse side of the coin and to gain a better understanding of what it is like to be a supervisor and what the role entails. This type of teaching/mentoring is certainly more intensive than providing tutorials, but if you have the opportunity to do this, you should take it! Not only will you learn new skills but also you will likely learn more about yourself and how you respond to a new leadership role.

12.4 Teaching at work

It is much easier to get involved in teaching when working at a hospital – such that it would be surprising to find someone who has worked in a hospital but not been involved in any teaching! This is especially true of tertiary centres and teaching hospitals. Again, this can take the form of formal or informal teaching opportunities.

Universities that send students to your particular hospital will always be looking for new people to teach their students. There may already be a formal teaching programme for students at your hospital. This may have a set schedule and topics; therefore, you simply need to reach out to the undergraduate management staff at your hospital, and they'll provide you with all of the information on how to get started. Where a teaching programme is not already established for students of your particular discipline, we strongly recommend you take the opportunity to set one up – this is not only an excellent way of getting teaching experience, it will also enrich your organisational and management skills. This can be done by reaching out to the undergraduate management staff for the universities that send students to your hospital and

Chapter 12

offering your services. Work collaboratively with them and the students to come up with a curriculum of topics that they want to be delivered to the students, and once you have these, you can canvass your fellow members of staff and request them to deliver teaching on those topics. You will also need to arrange suitable locations and times – we recommend lunchtime sessions in your hospital's education/academic centre. Students and teachers alike will prefer to teach at their usual site and during normal work hours, for convenience.

We would also recommend giving the teachers licence to decide whether or not they want to deliver the teaching session in a didactic format or do other things like deliver it by the bedside with real patients or even through simulation – a technique that has grown exponentially.

As a formal programme, it is important to get formal recognition from the university and use the undergraduate staff to help with organisation – including communication with the students regarding times and locations of sessions.

These principles also apply for teaching staff members. Postgraduate training programmes for medical and non-medical healthcare professionals have designated training days and curricula. We recommend that you also reach out to the programme directors or postgraduate staff to offer your services to provide teaching on your particular discipline/specialty. They will be delighted to hear from you, as, even if your topic lies outside the curriculum, they often have cancellations and gaps in their teaching rota, which they will be delighted to fill.

Case Study 12.4 Teaching in the workplace

As a junior doctor, I volunteered to be a faculty member of my hospital's simulation course for senior-year medical students. This involved delivering lectures on specific curriculum topics such as upper gastrointestinal bleeding and leading simulation sessions on these same topics. This had the double benefit of teaching me how to prepare focused PowerPoint lecture presentations and gaining experience leading simulation sessions.

This was an already established programme that had been running for years and allowed junior doctors rotating through the hospital to pass on their knowledge and experience to students coming behind them. The experience with simulation teaching was key in my obtaining an invitation, as a surgical trainee, to be a faculty member on a simulation course for London's surgical trainees. This is just an example of how taking one opportunity leads to other, higher-level opportunities.

Chapter 12

Informal teaching is at the foundation of postgraduate medical education. At all levels, healthcare professionals are expected to undertake work-based assessments. These include case-based discussions, clinical evaluation exercises, or directly observed procedures (DOPs). They serve as a mechanism for healthcare professionals to teach specific topics and procedures as well as provide immediate feedback to learners, including pointing out where they need to improve and highlight their progress. We recommend that you use these instruments to teach your juniors in hospital-specific topics, examinations, and procedures, as appropriate.

Informal teaching at work can take many guises; however, most common is in the form of bedside teaching. Students often appreciate and benefit from being shown how to perform specific clinical examinations on real patients in the clinical setting. This is particularly useful for students undergoing objective structured clinical examinations (OSCEs), in which they are observed carrying out clinical activities, for example, examining a patient with a painful knee.

Case Study 12.5 Informal teaching on the wards

As a surgical registrar, I used the instrument of 'case-based discussion' to teach junior doctors on several topics that will be relevant in their daily practice. An example of this was thyroid disease, where, on receiving a referral for a patient with a thyroid swelling, we discussed important aspects of the history, examination, investigation, diagnosis, and management of the patient. In a clinical setting, I would often bring my students to see patients in clinic, or on the wards to see patients with a thyroid swelling in order to hone their skills in examination of a neck lump. I first spoke to the patient and ensured he or she was happy to assist in the teaching of students, which patients are often delighted to do.

It is also important to prepare adequately so that you can identify the most important information you wish to impart to your students. These are essentially their learning objectives for your session, and you can then target your lesson to ensure you ask all of the relevant questions that will achieve each learning outcome. For example, in patients with thyroid overactivity (Graves' disease) who are taking certain treatment (Carbimazole), there is a risk of immune cell compromise and therefore a risk of fatal infections. This potential complication is of extreme importance, so add it to your learning objectives and make sure to question your students on it! Once your sessions have ended, you can send out the learning objectives lists to your students so they can ensure they focus on the appropriate material.

Chapter 12

12.5 Planning a lesson

It is helpful to be able to present your sessions in an appealing manner that facilitates your students' learning. In order to do this, we like to think about two factors: the audience and the objectives.

12.5.1 The audience
Think of the audience in terms of (and answer) the following questions:

- Whom are you teaching?
- At what level are they in their studies?
- What interests them?
- How will they be examined, if at all, on the subject?
- How motivated are they to learn what you are teaching them?

These are important to consider because at each level and in each discipline, the way of addressing learners' needs will likely differ. For example, the way you would present information to first-year medical students learning cardiac physiology is going to be different from the way you teach final-year medical students about congestive heart failure. It may be appropriate to teach the first-year students in a didactic manner through a lecture, particularly considering how they will be examined for the course (e.g. multiple-choice questions). However, the final-year students will likely be examined on how they interact with patients – asking appropriate questions and picking up on clinical examination signs; therefore, it is more appropriate to teach them using bedside tutorials where they interact with patients and practice these skills.

At the other end of the spectrum are those who are learning for clinical practice – they won't be examined at all, but what you teach them will form the basis of their practice – therefore, what you teach them needs to be practical as well as correct.

12.5.2 The objectives
Having identified your audience, you can ensure what you are teaching is relevant to them by deciding on a few easy-to-understand objectives.

Think of your objectives in terms of (and answer) the following questions:

- What specific knowledge are you looking to impart?
- Can you distil your objectives into a few lines max?
- Why are your objectives useful to your target audience?

Chapter 12

Use these objectives to create an overall structure of the session, potentially having them inform your headings and subheadings, as well as ensuring that the finer content you are presenting meets these objectives. It is advisable to present these at the start of your session, refer to each when discussing it during your session, and, finally, make them the basis of your takeaway points at the end of your session. This ensures that both you and your audience keep the objectives in your minds during the session and may help with retention.

Case Study 12.6 Teaching in clinical practice

As a Specialist Registrar Year 3 (ST3) in ENT, I was requested to teach emergency department doctors about how to manage common ENT presentations they might encounter during their practice in the emergency department. Using the questions above, I thought about the audience and the objectives. My audience was a group of highly motivated and educated doctors, interested in emergency presentations, who would not be examined on what I was teaching them but would use the knowledge in their day-to-day clinical practice.

I decided to focus on diseases related to the ear because this is a common and often misunderstood area. The objectives for the session, therefore, were to outline the common ear-related diseases likely to be seen in the emergency department. The first learning objectives were to discuss the common symptoms patients present with, i.e. what these doctors would see in their clinical practice. The second objective was to explain the best practice in the assessment of these patients in an emergency setting, and thirdly to discuss the emergency management of these conditions, i.e. what these doctors should do. The final objective was to highlight out common misconceptions relating to these conditions, i.e. what should not be done. By spending some time planning the session in this way, it was much easier to prepare my slides and, hopefully, much easier to engage the students and ensure the learning objectives were achieved. It is vital to tailor your teaching to each specific audience for maximum impact.

12.6 Getting the most out of your teaching

Whilst teaching is rewarding in itself, it gives you the opportunity to develop other skills and build up your CV. Here, we discuss how to maximise the return from your efforts.

12.6.1 Feedback

A key aspect of teaching is receiving feedback from the students you are teaching as well as your senior colleagues who have more teaching experience. Feedback from seniors should be collected both formally through work-based assessments and also informally. There are electronic forms available on online professional portfolios such as the Intercollegiate Surgical Curriculum Programme for surgical trainees. We recommend that you become acquainted with the appropriate portfolio for your discipline/specialty and look for mentors who are interested in teaching and who will be willing to observe you and provide formal feedback.

Where you don't have access to an electronic portfolio, paper forms are available online, which can be printed and used instead. Postgraduate management staff can also be helpful in directing you towards the best resources for your discipline in such a situation. The feedback can be used to bolster your professional portfolio, but a more prudent use is for the improvement of your teaching skills. Look at this feedback honestly and reflect on it – ask, frankly, how to improve, and try out the tips where appropriate. Senior colleagues have a wealth of information and teaching resources, tapping into which will only improve your experience.

Feedback from students is also valuable for the purposes of knowing what works well and what doesn't. We recommend, where possible, to gather this immediately after the teaching session, as it may be difficult to get responses at all, let alone accurate responses, from attendees days after the teaching session. Feedback forms can be found on specialty websites, e.g. the Royal College of Physicians. These are useful because they are standardised and reflect appropriate education standards for your specialty.

If you have the technical know-how and time, we recommend converting these into electronic format, e.g. via Google forms, and sending this form as a link to your students. It is useful to arrange in such a way that, once the attendees have returned feedback, they receive their attendance/completion certificate. This incentivises the returning of your feedback forms and enables you to keep soft copies for your portfolio.

Once you have the feedback, we recommend reflecting on it and writing a reflection for your portfolio. This is useful to improve your own teaching practice, and reflective practice is growing in use across healthcare disciplines, becoming increasingly recognised as a way to improve our practice.

12.6.2 Research

Whilst teaching and research are separate but essential disciplines in one's professional development, we have found that building research into your teaching can significantly enrich your experience. It is not always easy to build research into one's teaching, and it will, quite frankly, depend on what

Chapter 12

you are teaching and how you are teaching it – as some subjects and methods are more amenable to research than others. For example, it is relatively easy to build research into a teaching session where you are teaching a new skill or using a new method to teach – this can be done simply by measuring ability and/or confidence of the participants before and after the teaching session. You may even decide to use the captive audience of your students to research a separate, different topic, e.g. whilst teaching on one topic, you might take the opportunity to offer your students a survey on their attitudes and practice with regards to fluid and electrolyte prescribing or their experience with medical electives as students. We, therefore, recommend taking time to consider how you can build research into your teaching.

12.7 Running a teaching course

Running courses gives you the opportunity to develop your leadership and management skills, along with your teaching and research skills. It is a highly challenging prospect, which requires motivation, organisation, and considerable planning; however, it is massively rewarding, and the benefits far outweigh the cost of enduring the challenges. It also provides a big boost for your CV, with many specialty applications apportioning a significant number of points to applicants that have experience organising a relevant course. In some interviewing processes in the UK, teaching experience is more highly sought after than having an MSc or even a higher degree in clinical education. This reflects how multifaceted and challenging organising such a course can be.

For the purposes of this book, we have divided the courses you can run into novel and traditional. Traditional courses are ones that have been around for years, the content of which is centrally determined, e.g. by bodies such as Royal Colleges, and is delivered at multiple sites. An example of this is the Basic Surgical Skills course from the Royal College of Surgeons of England. A novel course, however, is your creation; you determine the content and deliver it at a site of your choice. Often it will be in response to a gap in the curriculum of a specialty or discipline with which you are familiar. There are multiple common facets in organising the two, thus experience and networks gained from one can be useful when embarking on organising the other.

12.8 How to set up a novel teaching course

Along with good planning and organisation, the key to a novel course is a good initial idea. How does one come up with such an idea? We've found that the best ideas are relevant to a particular discipline or specialty in which you are experienced, or at least very familiar. This gives you the insight to know what gaps there are in the curriculum and may give you a starting point on how to fill these gaps. We also recommend speaking to other people at various levels in your discipline or specialty and asking them specific questions about areas they feel are not covered by the curriculum or that they feel would benefit from extra coverage.

Once you have your idea, the next step is to define the problem as fully as possible and get objective data to support your endeavours. This will help later on when pitching the course to potential participants, and it is also a good opportunity to run a parallel research project.

For the first part it is best to focus your research on finding out the following:

1. Is there a problem? Are the majority of people in your discipline or area experiencing it?
2. What are the potential causes of the problem?
3. How might they be addressed?

A simple survey, using a free online tool like SurveyMonkey, can allow you to quickly gather data on the views and attitudes of your potential course attendees as well as useful information on content for your course.

We then encourage you to enlist the help of a senior person in your field, ideally someone with experience in running courses, be they novel or traditional courses. This is where the data you have collected comes in handy. You can show this to your senior colleague to aid you in enlisting his or her help – a colleague is much more likely to be convinced to help you if he or she sees the problem and how your course will help to address it, and input will be invaluable in allowing you to decide important practical factors:

- Duration of course.
- Course content.
- Format of delivery.
- Faculty.
- Venue.
- Resources required.
- Budget.
- Timetable.
- Recruitment of participants.

It is also useful to discuss with members of the education team at your workplace. Many hospitals have education fellows and simulation fellows as well as simulation leads who can prove to be very helpful, especially if you approach them early and show them your data that describes the problem.

Chapter 12

Once you have made all of these decisions and enlisted the appropriate help, you are ready to go! Make sure you collect feedback from participants, not only on each section of the course but also overall; this will help you to see if the course has made any impact into addressing the primary problem. This feedback will also help you with further iterations of the course, allowing you to improve the course to meet its objectives each time you run it.

Case Study 12.7 Medical elective suitcase

Towards the end of my medical studies at the University College Dublin, I had a discussion with a fellow student who shared some very negative experiences from her medical elective in Zambia. Her experiences were concerning, and I wondered if this was a common experience. As a junior doctor, I performed a literature review and conducted a survey of my peers by posting a short SurveyMonkey on a junior doctor Facebook group. This showed that concerning experiences on medical electives were relatively common. I presented these findings to my training programme director, a prominent vascular surgeon with a lot of experience running established and novel courses. She helped to suggest the best location at our hospital for a course as well as sharing strategies for recruiting students and giving me the contact details for the Medical Protection Society and Ethicon, who would help by providing some free materials for use at the course. I developed the curriculum for the course based on the initial research I had performed, mixing in a variety of teaching methods – lectures, small group discussions, skills workshops, and simulation. The input from our simulation lead and clinical teaching fellows was invaluable and allowed fine-tuning of these sessions in order to deliver the learning objectives as best as possible.

I then set about recruiting my fellow junior doctors to be faculty; this was a relatively easy task as I was able to get their buy-in by showing them the problem (research results) and its solution (course programme) as well as taking care to place them in an area that suited them – for example, those who had significant surgical experience and had completed the Basic Surgical Skills course were assigned to the surgical skills section.

I also had to coordinate the timetable with the faculty's schedules – because it was running on a workday, i.e. the most convenient day for medical students to attend, I had to ensure that certain sessions ran at certain times to allow certain faculty to be present at a time when they had a colleague covering them on the ward. We also ensured we had some 'substitute' colleagues available in case anyone was unwell or couldn't get away from the ward – in such a situation, the 'substitute' would be available to take over the session.

Once we had a date, location, programme, timetable, and faculty, I proceeded to recruit students from the cohort of St George's University London and King's College London medical students who were rotating through our hospital – a simple email with details of what the course was about was sufficient.

On the days we ran the course, we made sure to have faculty briefings to ensure everyone knew what they were doing and where, as well as having a dedicated timekeeper to ensure all aspects of the course ran according to time. I also delivered pre-course and post-course surveys to evaluate the impact the course had on the students. I then published research describing the problem, the course, and the results of the course.

12.9 How to run an established course

This is often easier than setting up your own course, as the curriculum and how the course should be delivered are already prescribed by the accrediting body. This, however, presents its own challenges, in particular, gaining permission to run the course and ensuring the course meets the exact standards of the accrediting body.

These are intertwined problems, as you will find that you will not be given permission to run the course unless you can prove that it will meet the prescribed standards. Very often you will find that the course has already been run in your hospital and that there is someone already in charge of putting it on – this is the person with whom to make friends and impress. We suggest reaching out, sharing your interest, and asking if you can help at all. Often courses run more than once a year, and if you show your interest and are helpful to the person in charge, he or she will often turn to you for help running the course. We advise being a student on the course first and then being a general helper in a subsequent iteration – which allows you to observe and learn how to ensure the course meets the appropriate standards – before organising the course yourself.

Where a course is yet to run at your hospital, the task is more difficult; however, getting in touch with the appropriate accrediting body after recruiting the help of an appropriately senior and experienced mentor to supervise you may help you to obtain approval to run the course. We advise carefully scrutinising the very often high standards to which the course must be run and thinking long and carefully – making plans and contingency plans, and running these by your mentor and others who have run this course in the past at other centres, before finalising a date. There is really no substitute for going on a course and helping someone else run it before endeavouring to run it yourself – this will give you invaluable insights and contacts.

Chapter 12

Chapter 13 **Conducting an audit**

13.1 What is clinical audit?

There is a popular saying in business management; 'What doesn't get measured, doesn't get managed'. Well, clinical audit is the process of measuring current clinical practice and comparing it to a set of established standards or guidelines – essentially, the current best practice appropriate for that discipline. The purpose is to measure how well you are meeting these standards and give insight on how to improve the quality you are delivering to patients and stakeholders. It is, therefore, a tool of quality improvement. Having this in your mind is key, in order to allow you to perform successful audits.

13.1.1 Audit cycle

The other key component to be aware of is that clinical audit is a continuous process, which is often termed the 'audit cycle'. This is because when you have the data telling you where you are falling short of a standard or guideline, you should use it to inform decisions on how to improve. Once you have made these improvements, a re-audit is undertaken, often termed 'closing the loop'. This allows you to tell whether or not your intervention has been successful and what further gains can be made to optimise the quality you deliver.

13.1.2 Benefits of audit

Audit is paramount to holistic healthcare practice, where quality can be a matter of life or death. It also allows you to use skills you've picked up along the way, including throughout this book, and apply them in your practice, thereby having a direct impact on the care your patients receive. While many of the skills used are similar, be aware that clinical audit is different from research. In research, you are looking for new information or testing a hypothesis – in audit, there is no hypothesis, and you are testing your practice against already established and adopted guidelines and standards. That is not

How to Succeed in Medical Research: A Practical Guide, First Edition.
Robert Foley, Robert Maweni, Shahram Shirazi, and Hussein Jaafar.
© 2021 John Wiley & Sons Ltd. Published 2021 by John Wiley & Sons Ltd.
Companion website: www.wiley.com/go/foley/succeed

to say that all data gathered in an audit cannot also be deemed research. However, this will not always be possible, and most audit projects don't provide new information suitable to answer a research question.

Clinical audits are also useful as a tool for showing your interest in a particular specialty, your interest in providing quality care, and your ability to collect, analyse, and act on data. As such, clinical audit is often a component of job applications, with points allotted for the number and quality of audits completed. Audit is now such an important part of healthcare that many organisations have a fully staffed clinical audit department, available to help you throughout the process – we recommend getting in touch with this department and finding out what resources they can provide.

13.1.3 Levels of audit

Audits can be done at various levels, broadly divided into locally and nationally. Local audits can be at various levels:

1. Departmental level – A hospital otorhinolaryngology department auditing how well they adhere to the nasal fracture management pathway.
2. Directorate level – A hospital planned care directorate auditing how often they adhere to seeing cancer referrals within 2 weeks.
3. Hospital level – A sepsis audit to see how often patients receive the initial sepsis management within a given timeframe.

National audits are often undertaken by a national body, usually doing this by setting up a central database into which local groups can enter their data. A good example of this is the National Emergency Laparotomy Audit performed by the Royal College of Anaesthetists in the UK, with the relevant data for each individual patient being entered into a central database by doctors at numerous participating hospitals across the country. This is more efficient than a national body going out and carrying out the audit themselves throughout the country; though the latter may be necessary, e.g. the National Health Service (NHS) in the UK has a Care Quality Commission (CQC), which is an independent regulator of NHS hospitals and periodically carries out audits of hospitals to ensure they are providing a level of care consistent with the national standard.

13.2 Conducting an audit

In this section, we'll give a brief but comprehensive treatment of the steps to undertaking a successful audit. These can be broken down into:

- Topic choice.
- Audit criteria.

Chapter 13

- Data collection.
- Results comparison.
- Feedback and discussion.
- Change implementation.
- Closing the loop and maintaining change.

13.2.1 Topic choice

Just like with research, the topic you choose can go a significant way in setting your audit up for success or failure. The ideal audit topic is one (i) in which you are interested, (ii) that makes an improvement in the experience of both patients and clinicians, (iii) that is clinically important, and (iv) that is financially important. Leaders of the organisation will tell you that they want you to audit a topic that is high priority for the organisation; the preceding list will often cover this, but you may also want to consider areas of high risks and high volume of work. This phase is also a good phase at which to select a supervisor for your audit – ideally someone who is experienced, approachable, and with whom you have a good rapport.

Following are a number of methods that might be useful at this phase.

13.2.1.1 What are you interested in?

Is there a particular niche in your discipline that interests you? A particular topic or condition you have come across that you found interesting? Answering these questions will give you a starting point on what topic to work on. Once you have a topic, e.g. vertigo, you can then look for guidelines in relation to the topic and consider which are most appropriate to audit.

13.2.1.2 What is not working for you and/or your patients?

The answer to this question is often an exasperated 'too many things!' However, we encourage you to dig deeper. Pick one thing – one factor, one aspect of your department – that could work better if the system around it were improved. We particularly like this method because it can have a real impact on the lives of your patients. That being said, it may also be worth auditing aspects of the department that are working well – this helps to prove that they are indeed working well or may identify further efficiencies to be gained.

13.2.1.3 Follow the money

What is costing your department or hospital the most? Can it be made more efficient? Saving your department money can make a big impact on your patient care – this saved money can be used to deliver better care to your patients in other areas.

13.2.1.4 Ask your seniors for suggestions
They have experience of what works as an audit and what doesn't work locally, and they will often be obliged to be involved in at least one audit per year for their continuing professional development. This approach, unfortunately, does carry the risk of you ending up doing an audit about a topic in which you are not particularly interested.

13.2.1.5 Take on an audit someone else has started
There are often audits started by someone else but not completed or at least in need of loop closing. You can find these out simply by contacting the local audit lead to ask if there are any in your department. This is a good opportunity to get some initial experience with audit and often involves less groundwork. We recommend getting in touch with the initial auditor and asking for any resources he or she may have, e.g. data collection tools. It is poor etiquette to re-audit someone else's work without first informing the person.

13.2.1.6 Contact the audit department
As well as information regarding previous audits, the audit department will have a list of audits that need to be done for your particular department at that time, and doing some of these is a good way to help your organisation.

There are often many aspects to each topic – many aspects to each guideline/protocol/standard; you don't need to audit all of them. You can just focus on and audit one aspect – this reduces the amount of work you need to do, but most importantly means that when you make an intervention, it will be more targeted and more likely to succeed.

Case Study 13.1 Surgical drain usage
As mentioned previously, you will not always have to start an audit from the beginning and may be able to complete an audit that a colleague has started. This was my experience in the following audit. As a medical student, I undertook an elective in neurosurgery at a London hospital. It just so happened that during my 2-week stint there, an audit meeting took place in which the results of an audit were presented. This audit looked at the rate of drain usage in surgery for patients with a 'bleed on the brain' (i.e. a subdural haematoma). There was randomised controlled trial evidence from supporting the use of a drain as part of this procedure. The use of a drain led to improved mortality and less recurrence of the subdural haematoma. The initial audit results demonstrated drain usage of 35%.

I returned to the same hospital as a junior doctor a few years later. I contacted the surgeon who was in charge of the audit I had seen and offered to help with a re-audit if this had not already been done. Luckily, it had not! The consultant was happy for me to perform the re-audit, and so I contacted the junior doctor who had performed the previous audit for advice and to discuss the project. I then contacted the administrative staff in the neurosurgery department to get a list of patients who had the operation in question since the previous audit. I read through each patient's operation note and simply recorded whether or not a drain was used. The use of a drain improved from 35% to 75% on the re-audit. This was a very easy task and not particularly time-consuming; following this, I presented the results to the neurosurgery department. The previous junior doctor who performed the initial audit was a very proactive individual, and once I had finished the re-audit, he took the lead on writing a paper and submitting it for publication. The paper, although not a research study, demonstrated that audit is an effective means of bringing the best clinical evidence into clinical practice.

Although not a huge amount of effort on my part, I was able to take part in an important audit that led to improvement and better outcomes for patients. This audit led to meaningful change and effectively coupled clinical practice and the latest evidence. I learned from this audit that published evidence in the literature is not enough to change practice. Whilst I had originally thought of publication as the end of a long research process, this is not the case. The dissemination of that research must continue afterwards in order to expose one's findings and lead to effective change.

13.2.2 Audit criteria

This is the process of deciding upon the most appropriate standards or guidelines to audit against. This should be a relatively easy part of the process – most departments will have established pathways/protocols/guidelines and standard operating procedures for commonly encountered clinical situations. Where there isn't any such local guideline, look for organisational and national guidelines. These should cover nearly every topic. Rarely would you need to look at international guidelines; however, these are often already adapted for local purposes.

Once you have done this, you should set the standard to which the practice is supposed to comply. This is often an optimum standard denoted by percentage, e.g. 100% compliance to a specific aspect of the protocol. Minimum standards can be appropriate in some situations, e.g. the NHS has a minimum standard that 85% of patients should start a first treatment for cancer within 2 months (62 days) of an urgent GP referral. Once you have your audit

---

Case Study 13.2 Outpatient clinic audit

As a junior doctor working in an ear, nose, and throat (ENT) department in the UK, one of my seniors felt they were seeing too many patients in the outpatient clinic. It transpired that our hospital didn't actually have a guideline stipulating how many patients should be seen in each clinic. However, the national body, ENT UK, had recently published guidelines stipulating how many patients should be seen by clinicians at each level during outpatient clinic – these were recommended for safety, and as such would have 100% standard. I, therefore, carried out an audit of the outpatient clinics over a period of 1 month and found that we had an overall compliance of 64%, and only 61% when we measured appropriate numbers of new patients being seen in each outpatient clinic session. This provides us with the appropriate data to make a change in our department, to ensure each patient is given adequate time to have his or her issues managed.

---

topic and criteria chosen, this is the time to register it with the audit department after discussion with your supervisor.

13.2.3 Data collection

The principles and practice of data collection are dealt with in detail in Chapter 2. However, there are a few important points with regards to clinical audit.

13.2.3.1 Amount of data/duration

We advise that you make sure the data you collect represents a long enough period to appropriately reflect the practice you are trying to measure. It will depend on the specific practice you are auditing and your setting – location, frequency of the phenomenon you're measuring, how easy it is to get data, etc. We, therefore, advise discussing data collection with your supervisor and coming to a reasonable conclusion that will capture the appropriate numbers of patients but not encumber you with unnecessary work.

13.2.3.2 Specificity of data

It is also prudent to think about what data you want to collect – make sure you collect data that you can directly compare to your guideline. It sounds easy, but it's even easier to collect data and then realise at a later stage that it's not complete – that it doesn't directly compare to your guideline. Take some time to really consider what data you should collect, and learn as you go along; you will often find that there are other criteria that you had not considered – don't hesitate to learn and incorporate these into your data collection process.

13.2.3.3 *Retrospective versus prospective*

We find the best way, given limited time, is to initially do a retrospective analysis to measure the results of current practice. This allows you to make an intervention based on the results and then audit the results of your intervention prospectively. However, retrospective data collection can have a variety of issues, including delays in getting patient notes and then the notes not containing the exact information you need.

13.2.4 Results comparison

This is the process of comparing your data against the standard that you have chosen. It's key to make sure you're comparing apples with other apples, rather than with oranges. Recall our earlier suggestion to audit only one aspect of a topic – this also helps you when it comes to analysis. By reducing the number of variables you measure, you reduce the number of variables you need to analyse, which also helps you to make sure you compare the appropriate factors. Be clear to compare your results against the appropriate minimum or optimum standard.

13.2.5 Feedback and discussion

This is a good opportunity to gain experience with presenting results of a study in a safe, local forum. The ideal place to do this is during a departmental meeting at which all (or at least most) of the stakeholders are in attendance – in medical teams, this may be in the form of a monthly clinical governance meeting. We advise you to make a PowerPoint/Keynote presentation with not just the results but also giving the context of the results. Whilst creating this – and thinking about your results – we recommend that you ask yourself, 'How can these results be improved?' It is good practice to include a suggested action plan in your presentation, and this will help you formulate an appropriate plan. Try to make your suggested actions SMART – specific, measurable, attainable, realistic and time-bound. This will make the next steps easier.

When you make your presentation, encourage discussion by members of your team and other stakeholders – particularly with a view towards giving suggestions for an action plan. Also invite discussion and feedback on the audit itself; be open to criticism here, as it will help you improve further audits and presentations and help with the re-auditing process.

13.2.6 Change implementation

This can, simultaneously, be the most exciting and most frustrating part of the audit process! It is well known that humans can be resistant to change, particularly change that requires different ways of working or added work for them. To successfully implement change, you need buy-in from all of the appropriate stakeholders – make sure you seek this in a tactful way. It could be as simple as convincing colleagues at your level to do something differently or as complex as requiring changes to electronic systems; either way, you need to convince those involved that helping you, though potentially increasing their workload temporarily, will ultimately benefit the organisation and patients. This is a bit easier if the change you want to carry out has been approved at the discussion meeting, and the people who are going to carry it out have contributed to its conception.

13.2.7 Closing the loop and maintaining change

Once you have implemented the plan, it is important to measure the effects of the change with another audit. We recommend doing this prospectively – it's much easier and allows you to see the progress, giving insight into how you can potentially improve it going forward. Repeat all of the above steps, learning and making improvements to deliver quality. You can also maintain change by handing over the audit to someone else – ideally someone who is a permanent fixture in the department/organisation, who has bought into the idea and is in a position to drive further improvements. It is also important to be aware that guidelines can change over time, and they often have to be reviewed after a certain period of time – why not volunteer to be on the panel in charge of reviewing the guideline against the latest research?

Case Study 13.3 Medical management of miscarriage audit

As a junior doctor rotating in obstetrics and gynaecology (O&G) at a London hospital, I noticed that a significant proportion of patients admitted for medical management of miscarriage failed this treatment option and therefore, progressed to surgical management. I wondered why this was happening and carried out an audit of the local protocol. Medical management was based around the use of a medication called misoprostol, which is inserted into the vagina. A protocol for this clinical situation was available within the obstetrics department, and this was taken as the gold standard.

The results of the initial audit demonstrated that our success rate with medical management of miscarriage was only 61% – significantly below the internationally noted success rate of 80–90%. We also found that there was inconsistency in the prescribing practices; with the appropriate doses of misoprostol not always being prescribed for the appropriate gestation age. This led me to wonder if this was contributing to the low rate of successfully managed miscarriage.

I also found that only 40% of patients had regular painkillers prescribed and that only 60% of patients had painkillers prescribed as required. This was

Chapter 13

important because this is a painful experience for the patients and is one of the reasons why they require admission to hospital – to control their pain. The inconsistent prescribing practice was likely because junior doctors responsible for prescribing the protocol were rotating through the specialty over a period of 4 months, and the variance in prescribing practice may well be due to a lack of awareness of the protocol.

As part of my investigation into the results of the survey, I also conducted a survey of the nursing staff to ascertain their practice and experience. I found that none of them had prior education of misoprostol administration and only 8% administered the misoprostol into the posterior fornix of the vagina, which is where it is more likely to be retained and have a full effect. Indeed, 33% of nurses had found the misoprostol external to the vagina when checking on their patients.

After presenting and discussing my findings with the department head, we initiated some interventions:

- Education of medical staff and nurses.
- Up-to-date protocol to be placed on the ward, in an easy-to-access location.
- Poster with clear and simple instructions placed in the doctor's office, the nurse's station, and the utility room.

These were cheap and easy interventions and had significantly improved all the outcome measures when I re-audited the department. With this loop closed and all measures improved, I then sought to improve efficiency in the system. My next intervention was to take advantage of the hospital's electronic prescribing system to create a button to select 'Medical Management of Miscarriage Orderset', in which doctors would only need to select the appropriate gestational age and the correct drugs and doses would be automatically selected for the patient. This would ensure 100% adherence to the prescription aspect of the protocol and hopefully improve the number of patients successfully treated medically.

However, I was then rotating to a different hospital, and therefore I handed the project over to two new Foundation year 1 doctors who were starting their O&G rotations as I was leaving. I also ensured to get buy-in from the electronic prescribing system's lead pharmacist, who was a permanent staff member at the hospital and would be key to ensuring the changes were implemented correctly. The obstetrics department was able to maintain the change and continue to improve long after I left the hospital. This case study illustrates how to actively engage with the audit process and to make lasting change in your workplace.

Remember the saying 'What doesn't get measured, doesn't get managed' and think about where you can start making an impact in your organisation.

Chapter 14 **Portfolio/CV**

14.1 Keeping a portfolio

Right from the start of your career in healthcare, you will be required to maintain a portfolio of all of your achievements. This may be a certificate from courses you attend, copies of any work assessments you undertake, quality improvement programmes you carry out, or any reflections you compose. These are essential to perform throughout your training or employment; however, it is also essential that you keep evidence of everything you have done. Take the opportunity to invest in an A4 folder and develop a physical paper portfolio of your work.

There are a number of important sections to include in your portfolio, including those in the following example:

- Table of contents.
- An up-to-date copy of your CV.
- Undergraduate and postgraduate degree certificates.
- Additional qualifications.
- Academic course certificates.
- Audits and quality improvement projects (QIPs).
- Record of teaching experience.
- Presentations.
- Conferences attended.
- Publications.
- Evidence of leadership and management positions.
- Evidence of commitment to your specialty – in the case of a doctor in training, for example, you may have membership of a relevant society, a clinical or operative logbook, or a letter confirming attendance at a taster session.

How to Succeed in Medical Research: A Practical Guide, First Edition.
Robert Foley, Robert Maweni, Shahram Shirazi, and Hussein Jaafar.
© 2021 John Wiley & Sons Ltd. Published 2021 by John Wiley & Sons Ltd.
Companion website: www.wiley.com/go/foley/succeed

- Additional achievements, both academic or extra-curricular.
- Additional reflections.

Depending on your career path, a paper portfolio may even be a mandatory requirement of any interview process. It is important to start early and update your portfolio on a frequent basis to ensure it includes a record of all of the work you have carried out to date. Collating evidence for your portfolio from scratch takes a lot of time and organisation. If you have yet to start your portfolio, do so as soon as possible and well in advance of any interviews.

It may seem daunting to ask supervisors or senior colleagues to provide evidence of your involvement in a project, but they will have been through a similar process themselves and appreciate it is something you need to help you progress your career. Try to ask for a letter as soon as possible after a project is completed. Find out who the secretary is and send an email to both your supervisor and his or her secretary, along with details of the project you worked on, and remind them of your role in it. If you do not hear back from them after a while, don't give up, send a polite reminder or ask them if they would prefer to schedule in some time with you so they can write the letter with you present. If you are currently in work, try to track down any awards or achievements from your time in undergraduate or postgraduate education. The best person to contact about these would be the course administrator or a member of administrative staff for your course.

As you may need to show the contents of your portfolio to an interview panel, you should organise your portfolio in a structured way. Research the exact requirements and lay out your portfolio in the order they have suggested.

Here are a few little tips on making things easy to find in your portfolio:

- Use dividers and write the section name on each one.
- Create a contents page for each individual section.
- Include additional tabs and highlighters where necessary to draw the interviewer's attention to specific areas.
- Order your portfolio within each subsection to prioritise the evidence that is the most important and most likely to impress the interviewers.

If you have been involved in audits or publications, create a summary page and tabulate your achievements by project. For audits or QIPs, include the name and date of the project, your exact role, whether the audit loop is open or closed, and if you subsequently presented the project. For publications, include the name and date of the publication, the journal it was published in, and your exact role. Summarising your work in this manner will make it easy for interviewers to find the information they need and make you look organised.

Case Study 14.1 Audit Section

It is important to be neat, organised, and systematic when laying out your portfolio to help you find the evidence you need easily but also to allow anyone looking through your portfolio to find the important information immediately and to understand where everything is located if they wish to delve deeper into a particular section. The audit section of my portfolio begins with a contents page, which outlines the page number and what each page of the portfolio demonstrates. The first page consisted of a summary table, like so:

Audit	Role	Audit cycle	Presentation	Date
Assessing Use of Thromboembolic Deterrent Stockings in Croydon University Hospital	Audit lead	Closed loop	Regional	November 2018
DVT Prophylaxis in Colorectal Cancer Patients – NICE Guideline CG92	Contributor	Closed loop	Regional	December 2016
Review of Ward-Based Care – UK Working Party for Acute Pancreatitis Patients Guidelines	Audit lead	Open loop	Local	July 2018
"? Obstruction" – Compliance with Royal College of Radiology iRefer Guidelines for Requesting Abdominal Plain Films	Audit lead	Open loop	Local	March 2018
Outcomes After Acute Kidney Injury in Surgery (OAKS 1)	Site lead (multicentre audit)	Open loop	—	January 2016

Next, for each audit, I included the following:

- An audit summary, including my exact contribution to each project.
- Abstract (200–250 words).
- Copy of poster or slides from an oral presentation.
- Letter or certificate confirming role in project.
- Personal reflection on what I learned in the process.

Although this is quite a lot of work to do, it will demonstrate your organisational skills and your ability to learn from your projects, specifically when a personal reflection is included.

Chapter 14

Case Study 14.2 Academic Courses Section

The academic courses section of your CV is an opportunity to really stand out. Although lots of courses will have been taken by your peers and will be common to everyone's portfolio, the inclusion of a reflection on each academic course is a chance to go that extra step. We recommend including a reflection for each course you have attended. Here is an example reflection for the Advanced Trauma Life Support (ATLS) course created by the American College of Surgeons:

PERSONAL REFLECTIVE LOG: *ATLS (11–12 September 2018)*

What were the key issues covered and the learning benefits noted?
- Systematic assessment and management of a trauma patient using ATLS A-E algorithm
- Understanding of the purposes of primary and secondary survey and familiarity with performing these
- Team working during a trauma call and appreciation of different roles

What can I put into practice immediately by way of an action plan?
- Partake in trauma calls in A&E

What can I put into practice over the medium to long term by way of an action plan?
- Book additional courses such as CCRISP to further improve clinical skills and Knowledge
- Utilise ATLS knowledge to teach surgical junior doctors by doing case based discussions and carry out simulation teaching

What further reading / research could I do?
- Further reading on surgical management of trauma patients

Figure 14.1   An example reflection.

We would encourage you to complete these shortly after attending the course, using the same headings we have above or your own if you feel they are more appropriate. Print your reflection and place it in your portfolio immediately next to your course attendance certificate. Reflecting in this way not only demonstrates to interviewers that you are actively thinking about what you learned on the course but it will also genuinely help you to consolidate your learning. It will allow you to increase your awareness of your limitations and identify your future learning needs and how to implement what you have learned to improve yourself, rather than merely collecting a certificate.

Chapter 14

14.2 Curriculum vitae (CV)

Your CV is a concise record of all of your achievements to date. It is essentially the same as your portfolio without the evidence! It will consist of similar sections as a portfolio and will list your achievements in each section. A sample CV of one of the authors has been included in the online content section that accompanies this book.

The sections included in our sample CV are:

- Your particulars/details.
- Education
  ○ This is a list of my academic qualifications.
- Radiology Experience
  ○ This has a separate section as it is my chosen medical specialty.
- Clinical Experience
  ○ In this section I outline my working life thus far.
- Student Electives
  ○ This is a list of my clinical and research electives as a medical student.
- Foundation Taster Sessions
  ○ These are short stints during my working life, in which I spent time in other departments within hospitals to gain experience.
- Academic Courses
- Publications
  ○ We illustrate how to display your publications in the upcoming Case Study 14.3.
- Abstract Publications
  ○ These may be all publications or a selection of the most important ones.
- Audit Experience
- Formal Teaching Experience
  ○ Include any formal teaching positions you held, such as an honorary tutor, etc.
- Leadership and Management Experience
- Awards and Honours
- Presentations
  ○ These can be split into poster and oral/podium presentations.
- Peer Review Experience

Case Study 14.3 Publications Within Your CV

A full sample CV is available to look through in the online content section; however, we will illustrate here an example of how to present publications within your CV. Make sure the publications are easy to read and separated out by newest to oldest. Some key points are to make sure you highlight your own position within the authorship, which can be done as shown in Figure 14.2. It is also important to include a PubMed identification number, if you can, to demonstrate that the publication is indexed on PubMed. The DOI (Digital Object Identifier) is a unique number assigned to each publication and allows your article to be easily located.

PUBLICATIONS

1. **Maweni RM,** Shirazi S, Chatzoudis D, Das S; *Laryngocoele*   2018
   *with contralateral laryngopyocoele – rare case of respiratory
   distress;* BMJ Case Reports; September 2018;
   DOI: 10.1136/bcr-2018-225444; **Pub Med ID**: 30181400

2. **Maweni RM,** Foley RW, Lupi M, Woods A, Shirazi S, Holm V,   2018
   Vig S; *Improving safety for medical students and patients
   during medical electives – a novel simulation based course;*
   Irish Journal of Medical Science; 29 October 2018;
   DOI: 10.1007/s11845-018-1919-6; **Pub Med ID**: 30374800

3. Lupi M, **Maweni RM,** Shirazi S, Umar JW; *Fluid and Electrolyte*   2018
   *Balance-Establishing the knowledge base of Foundation Year
   One Doctors;* Irish Jounal of Medical Science;
   DOI: Pending – in Press; **Pub Med ID**: Pending – in Press

Present your publications in this format, ensuring to highlight your own name to draw attention to your role, and include a PubMed ID if you have one.

Figure 14.2 An example of CV publication presentation.

Chapter 15 **Maintaining a good balance**

There is nothing either good or bad, but thinking makes it so. . .
Hamlet, William Shakespeare, 1608.

Working in healthcare can be incredibly rewarding. The combination of making a difference to patients' lives through clinical work and undertaking scientific research and other academic pursuits, in our opinion, provides a fulfilling experience that is very difficult for any other profession to match.

The nature of the decisions we make, compounded with the long working hours and the challenges of working in under-pressure healthcare systems, can all take a toll on your physical and mental well-being. This can be even more challenging if you want to pursue scientific research alongside your clinical work.

We have often wished universities offered modules on preparing students for the biopsychosocial impact of doing the job for which they are studying, rather than only focusing on such core subjects as anatomy and physiology. However, we have found that, though many universities don't have specific modules on this, the process of going through university – meeting the various deadlines, passing the examinations, and maintaining social relationships along the way – helps to develop strategies and habits that many carry into the workplace. While some of these are helpful, they are not always ideal for the workplace, and indeed there are other factors that prevent them from being effective.

Think about it – staying up late the night before an important assignment is due may work in university, but is it likely to work when you're working a night shift before a key abstract submission deadline?

In this chapter, we offer some advice on how to stay happy at work and to maintain a healthy balance in your work and personal life. It is, however, important to be aware that the contents of this chapter are by no means

How to Succeed in Medical Research: A Practical Guide, First Edition.
Robert Foley, Robert Maweni, Shahram Shirazi, and Hussein Jaafar.
© 2021 John Wiley & Sons Ltd. Published 2021 by John Wiley & Sons Ltd.
Companion website: www.wiley.com/go/foley/succeed

exhaustive, and those strategies that might work for one person may not work for another. We, therefore, encourage you to try to learn what works for you – take time to think about it and find the appropriate strategies for yourself early in your career, and this will make life much easier for you.

15.1 Stress and burnout

Stress occurs when an individual feels that the demands required of him or her exceed the capacity to cope with those demands. It is a common occurrence in healthcare professionals. Often the cause of stress is multifactorial, and it can be related to work colleagues, patients, healthcare systems and structures, or a number of other factors. Stress may be caused by something outside of work but exacerbated by work pressures. Burnout is the end stage of stress. It occurs when we are unable to keep up with the pressures being placed on us over a period of time. Many people can have a stressful day but then not let this affect them too much, and they bounce back to a positive mindset the following day. But few will be able to deal with a stressful work life on a chronic basis without some sort of psychological impact.

There are a number of ways to notice when you are feeling stressed or burned out, if you are not already aware that you have this problem. Stress can manifest with physical symptoms such as headaches, behavioural symptoms such as anger, or emotional symptoms such as excessive worrying. Are you acting with anger at work? This can manifest in obvious ways, such as shouting at colleagues, or be more subtle and demonstrated by us taking less interest in other people's points of view in conversation. We may also start to interrupt others, tend to criticise, be resentful of other people's actions, or be quick to blame others. Burnout can also often manifest as disinterest. Have you become less interested in your job? Do you feel as if what you do is no longer important or worth doing? The first step towards dealing with these issues is to become aware of them.

If you are feeling angry, stressed, burned out, or overwhelmed, seek help! There are a number of resources available. These include self-help books and websites or formal supports via your hospital/university or your own doctor. Following are some practices you may find helpful.

15.1.1 Take a timeout

This is particularly helpful when feeling angry or overwhelmed. Take a moment to separate yourself from the situation. If you are becoming angry while talking to colleagues, tell them you can no longer continue at this point, but you will continue your conversation with them later. And then leave the situation. You will find this enables you to think more clearly before responding, and you will often change both the message you were trying to convey and the method of conveying it.

15.1.2 Focus on the positives
Try to focus on your people skills and having positive interactions with others. This will allow you to remain empathetic.

15.1.3 Realise that you are not perfect
Perfectionist thinking is a common 'thought error' we can make, and deeming ourselves a failure if we are not perfect goes hand in hand with this. Realising that we are not perfect can open ourselves up to feeling better. Do your best, and be proud of what you have achieved whilst doing your best!

15.1.4 Mindfulness meditation and self-compassion meditation
These methods can allow us to calm down, to give our minds some peace and time to refuel. Mindfulness calls on us to focus on the present moment, while self-compassion can allow us to comfort ourselves, to recognise that we are suffering, and to feel loved.

15.1.5 Breaks
Avoid working for long periods of time without a break or breathing space. You can use this time to do something you enjoy, like listening to your favourite song.

15.1.6 Stress log
Try to keep a record of when you feel stress over the course of a week, both at work and at home. This may help you to find some of the triggers for your stress and work out methods to avoid them.

Case Study 15.1 Burnout in the workplace

This topic is very close to my heart, and it is particularly important to talk about it openly and honestly. I have suffered with stress and burnout at work; however, I have also overcome it. When working my first year as a junior doctor, I was working a long weekend over Christmas, with four 13-hour shifts from Friday to Monday. I found these shifts incredibly difficult. We were understaffed, and essentially I was responsible for approximately 100 patients on the wards.

I had a horrendous experience over the course of this long weekend, and it culminated in my breaking down in tears on the ward on Christmas Day. I was emotional for the rest of the day, crying at a number of points, and over the subsequent weeks I found myself welling up at work quite frequently. There was too much work for me to handle on my own, and I allowed myself to become overwhelmed. This led to a feeling of severe burnout and withdrawal over the next few weeks. I found myself not caring about anything that happened while at work, and a number of my colleagues remarked at how angry I seemed to be. There was a definite change in my demeanour, and I hated coming to work over this time period.

I found it very difficult to deal with what I deemed as failure, and especially knowing that I had no one to help me, I felt completely lost. I was feeling helpless and annoyed at the ridiculous situation I was left in. As mentioned previously, this experience left me in a bad state for a number of weeks afterwards.

Over the next few weeks, I had the chance to think about what happened and reflect. I realised that I needed help, and I turned to an online cognitive behavioural therapy course for support. I was guilty of lots of self-deprecation and warped thinking; in particular, I was being a perfectionist and labelling myself a failure if I wasn't performing perfectly. I also began to read about mindfulness meditation, and I started to incorporate these practices into my daily routine and drew up mindfulness when I was becoming stressed at work.

On my next long stint of weekend shifts, I also instigated a number of changes at work to help me. Firstly, I made an attitudinal adjustment. I made a conscious effort not to become overwhelmed with the workload and to try to stay relaxed and composed. Secondly, I made practical changes. I carried a wireless on-call phone with me for the weekend so that I could return bleeps/pages from the wards without running around looking for a phone. This meant that I could quickly deal with issues and not have to be bleeped/paged on multiple occasions. I also made a deliberate effort to work slower, making sure I finished one task before moving on to another. Avoiding trying to do too many things at once actually made me more efficient.

I also attempted to delegate tasks where possible, asking the nursing staff and other colleagues for help. Not doing this enough was largely the cause of much of my stress previously. These changes allowed me to have a much more manageable weekend and avoid the emotional turmoil I had previously experienced.

Stress at work and feelings of burnout can be difficult to avoid. The first step is recognising you are suffering, at which point you need to make the necessary steps to get help and improve your situation rather than let the negative emotions control you. I hope firstly that you will never have to suffer too severely from this, but if you do, I hope this case study will help you to remove yourself from it!

15.2 Improving your mindset to promote resilience

Josh Kaufman, author of the bestselling book The Personal MBA, coined the term 'Caveman Syndrome' to describe the fact that human biology is still optimised for the lifestyle that existed thousands of years ago rather than today's world [1]. 'Your brain and body simply aren't optimised for today's world'. It is optimised for a time when you had to conserve energy in order to escape from predators as well as hunt and gather for a living. While we can trace the increasing prevalence of lifestyle diseases such as diabetes mellitus to this fact, it can also help us understand why it might be difficult for us to sustain a life of working 13-hour day shifts, interspersed with 13-hour night shifts and occasional 8-hour work days – you simply weren't made to live that way. Such a lifestyle is sure to lead to burnout and significant biopsychosocial consequences – including depression, anxiety, and weight gain. And yet, this is a lifestyle many will be expected to live during their formative years as healthcare professionals. In fact, it has been reported that over half of doctors and almost as many other healthcare professionals in the US experience burnout [2].

One way of tackling this, in our opinion, is to build up your professional resilience. This is your ability to face and respond to high pressure and demand situations and to 'bounce back' when you face a setback. While there are many ways of doing this, we believe that improving your mindset is one key skill to possess.

15.2.1 Mindset

Stanford professor of psychology Carol Dweck has spent the past 30 years investigating how our beliefs, conscious and subconscious, impact our lives. Through the course of this research, she has found that humans have two main ways of looking at the world, two main mindsets, namely fixed and growth [3].

A fixed mindset is one whereby holders believe that their abilities and experiences in a particular domain (sometimes all domains) are static – they either have it or they don't – and they can't change or improve in any meaningful way. For people with such a mindset, challenges are an insurmountable obstacle.

In contrast, a growth mindset is one where holders believe that their abilities and experiences are malleable – that they can grow with training and effort. In this mindset, challenges are a means by which one can grow and improve his or her abilities.

Dweck has shown (and we have found in our own lives) that realising this, evaluating your mindset as it relates to important domains in your life, and then adjusting it where necessary to a growth mindset can lead to you improving your experiences in those domains. This is important in healthcare where we face many challenges – challenges that we can either see as insurmountable or as a means for our growth.

Chapter 15

Case Study 15.2 A growth mindset

As a surgical trainee, I was faced with challenges many face when they reach a new, higher level in their careers and lives. I was going from a level at which I was comfortable and could complete tasks efficiently to a new level where I had no experience. I knew I would encounter a steep learning curve to get back to the point where I felt comfortable and efficient again. After a couple of months of struggling to improve my operating skills, I decided to evaluate my mindset. I found that whilst I had a growth mindset about my training in general, I had a significantly fixed mindset about my abilities in regard to my surgical skills. I had fixed mindset beliefs such as

- I am naturally good or bad at certain procedures and can't meaningfully change that (blaming circumstances beyond my control).
- Some procedures are too difficult for me to do at my current level (blaming circumstances beyond my control).
- My trainer isn't interested in helping me (blaming others).

Realising this, and that I was getting in the way of my own progress, I set about actively changing my beliefs. Actively telling myself that I could improve and grow and all I needed to do was put in the effort – reading as much as possible, watching as many procedures as possible, and practicing my skills in these procedures as much as possible – was essential to overcoming my fixed mindset.

In a short space of time, my trainer told me I had made an 'exponential improvement' in my skills, but even before that, my enjoyment and understanding had grown so significantly that I was motivated to keep learning more. This is the difference your mindset can make.

15.3 Other methods for resilience

There are a number of other methods to build up your resilience so that you are not so badly affected by stress or burnout but also so that you have methods of relaxing and de-stressing after difficult days.

15.3.1 Passion projects

This is an activity you carry on, usually in your free time, because you enjoy it. The concept originates from film and television, but it can be adapted to mean any project that you do for enjoyment rather than only for financial gain. We recommend having such a project, in or outside work. What you choose to do should be based on your interests and what is available to you – but most of all, it should be an enjoyable distraction. Examples are myriad, but include learning an instrument, painting, starting a food blog, or car restoration. Indeed, in our more junior years as doctors, our research projects were all passion projects as well!

> **Case Study 15.3 AfroEights**
> I have always had an interest in video games – having spent 9 of the first 11 years of my life in a rural village in the Kalahari Desert in Botswana, video games were often the only source of entertainment. As a junior doctor, I started to learn how to develop games and learn some basic coding principles. In my spare time, I used these principles to develop a video game, which was an online version of a popular card game, Crazy Eights. I created an online multiplayer version of this game using the rules of the game as played in Africa. I thoroughly enjoyed this game, and when I shared it with others, I found they enjoyed it too, such that I have had to make it publicly available to be down-loaded under the name 'AfroEights'.

15.3.2 Health

We have often found, when speaking to other healthcare professionals, that they put the health of their patients and others above their own. While this may sound counter-intuitive (who will help those people if you become so unwell you can't function?), it is very common and manifests itself in even more counter-intuitive behaviour, e.g. doctors and nurses turning up for work whilst sick and potentially spreading the illness.

We encourage you to put your health first. This goes for both your physical and emotional health, with the latter often being ignored and suffering as a result, directly contributing to burnout. Keeping habits that help to keep you in a healthy state is, therefore, helpful. Simple things like getting regular exercise, ensuring you take an appropriate number of meals per day, and getting enough sleep will go a long way towards keeping you well. See 'Practical Tips' below for more.

15.3.3 Relationships

Relationships in and outside the workplace are crucial in building up your resilience.

Good relationships can provide support and advice at key times, allowing you to share positive and negative experiences and continue to grow from them. Making friends in the workplace also allows you to take advantage of

Chapter 15

networking benefits and make your work easier – for instance, friends can show you how to do things more efficiently and effectively as well as helping you to share the load when needed. Make sure to invest time in the relationships that mean the most to you, both in work and outside work.

15.4 Practical tips

Taking care of yourself is paramount, and the following are a few tips we hope will help you in your career in healthcare.

15.4.1 Organise
Try to be organised and efficient with your work day. But also, try to be organised with your finances – make a budget and save. You can save for a target that is important to you, such as a holiday you have planned, which can serve as excellent motivation. Organise your work and personal life by keeping a calendar to remind you of important dates.

15.4.2 Be realistic
Leave work on time if you can. Medicine never sleeps. . .but you need to! There will always be more work that you can do, but that doesn't mean that you should stay up all night to do it! Hand over any urgent tasks to the on-call team and make a list of the non-urgent jobs for the next day. If there are too many for you to do, find others who can help.

15.4.3 Seek help
Work as a team as much as possible, delegate simple tasks to your juniors, ask for help with tasks you find difficult, and escalate problems to your seniors when you feel out of your depth.

15.4.4 Decompress
Take regular breaks throughout the day, a moment that is just yours to enjoy. Be sure to take a lunch break during the day and recharge. No matter how much work is waiting for you, it is important to be fed, watered, and prepared for work.

15.4.5 Socialise
Make time to meet your old friends but also make an effort to socialise with your current work colleagues and make new friends too!

References

1. Kaufman, J. (2012). *The Personal MBA: A World-Class Business Education in a Single Volume*, 1e. London: Penguin.
2. Reith, T. (2018). Burnout in United States healthcare professionals: a narrative review. *Cureus* **10** (12): e3681. https://www.ncbi.nlm.nih.gov/pmc/articles/PMC6367114.
3. Dweck, C. (2017). *Mindset: Changing the Way You Think to Fulfil Your Potential*, 6e. London: Robinson.

Index

Note: Page numbers in *italic* refer to figures. Page numbers in **bold** refer to tables.

How to Succeed in Medical Research: A Practical Guide, First Edition.
Robert Foley, Robert Maweni, Shahram Shirazi, and Hussein Jaafar.
© 2021 John Wiley & Sons Ltd. Published 2021 by John Wiley & Sons Ltd.
Companion website: www.wiley.com/go/foley/succeed